The Herbal Remedies Medicine Bible

The Ultimate Collection of Healing Herbs and Plants. Use the Power of Alkaline Herbs to Detoxify your Organs, boost Immunity and restore Health

By

Elizabeth T. Rupert

Table of Contents

Introduction

Fundamentals of Herbalism

Welcome to the comprehensive guide to herbalism: a valuable resource for learning how to grow, use, and benefit from the extraordinary properties of medicinal plants. Herbalism has a long history of use in supporting human health and well-being, making it one of the oldest forms of medicine in the world.

To begin, we will explore the fundamental principles of herbalism. We will discover key terms and concepts used in this field, such as infusions, decoctions, herbal teas, ointments, and tinctures. Additionally, we will discuss the importance of following necessary precautions to ensure safe and effective use of medicinal plants.

Collecting Medicinal Plants Ethically

An essential part of herbalism is the ethical and sustainable collection of medicinal plants. We will learn how to recognize and properly identify plants, along with providing guidelines for respectful harvesting of plants to preserve the environment and natural resources. Furthermore, we will explore methods for preserving the collected plants to maintain their beneficial properties.

Preparing the Soil and Creating Your Medicinal Herb Garden

Before cultivating medicinal plants, it is crucial to prepare the soil adequately. We will explore how to choose the ideal site for our medicinal herb garden and how to prepare the soil for planting. Additionally, we will discuss the best arrangements and designs to optimize plant growth.

Cultivating Medicinal Plants

In this chapter, we will explore plants suitable for our needs and climate, providing detailed steps for successful sowing and transplanting of medicinal plants. We will also learn how to care for the plants during their growth period to ensure robust and healthy growth.

Harvesting, Drying, and Preserving

Once the plants have grown, it is time to harvest and prepare them for future use. We will see when is the best time to harvest medicinal herbs and how to properly dry them to preserve their therapeutic properties. Moreover, we will learn how to store the dried herbs to use them as needed.

Using Medicinal Plants

We arrive at the most exciting part of herbalism: using medicinal plants to prepare therapeutic remedies. We will provide you with recipes and detailed instructions for making infusions, decoctions, herbal teas, ointments, and tinctures. Additionally, we will explore specific remedies for common ailments like colds, headaches, and muscle pains.

In-Depth Exploration and Integrations

In this chapter, we will delve into specific herbal traditions, such as Chinese or Ayurvedic medicine, to discover how medicinal plants are used in different cultures. Furthermore, we will explore how to integrate herbalism into everyday life, using medicinal plants in cooking, skincare, and more.

Herbalism for Children

Dedicated to the safe and appropriate use of medicinal plants for little ones, this chapter will offer advice for using herbal remedies to treat common childhood issues, such as stomachaches or colds.

Herbalism in Everyday Life

We will explore how to integrate herbalism into our daily lives to enhance overall well-being. Discover how to use medicinal plants in cooking, skincare, and creating household products.

Specific Remedies with Medicinal PlantsWe will furher explore the treatment of specific conditions using medicinal plants. Learn how to address headaches, insomnia, digestive disorders, and more.

Herbalism and Traditional Medicine

We will explore the integration of herbalism with traditional medicine and alternative medical practices, understanding how these different disciplines can work together for individual well-being.

We will conclude this guide to cultivating and using medicinal plants, reflecting on the significance of herbalism for health and well-being. We will encourage readers to continue their learning journey in herbalism and deepen their knowledge of medicinal plants.

With this structure, the book covers a wide range of topics and delves into each aspect of herbalism, offering readers a comprehensive and detailed guide to cultivating and using medicinal plants safely and effectively.

Welcome to the fascinating world of herbalism. In this chapter of nature's remedies meets the wisdom of ancient healing traditions. In this chapter we will embark on a journey to explore the fundamental relationship between plants and [...]

A solid understanding of this topic is essential for anyone wishing to harness the incredible potential of nature's pharmacy for health and well-being.

1.1 What is Herbalism?

At its core, herbalism is the practice of using plants and their extracts to promote health, prevent illness, and to treat various ailments. Its roots stretch back to the earliest chapters of human civilization, when our ancestors first learned to identify and utilize the healing properties of the plants that surrounded them. Today, herbalism continues to thrive, offering a natural approach to health and wellness.

1.2 Key Terminology

To truly understand the world of herbalism, it is essential to become familiar with some of its key terms and concepts. Here are a few of the most important that you will encounter.

17

Chapter 1: Fundamentals of Herbalism

Welcome to the fascinating world of herbalism, where the power of nature's remedies meets the wisdom of ancient healing traditions. In this chapter, we will embark on a journey to explore the fundamental principles that underpin the art and science of herbal medicine. By gaining a solid understanding of these key concepts, you will be better equipped to harness the incredible potential of medicinal plants for your health and well-being.

1.1 What is Herbalism?

At its core, herbalism is the practice of using plants and their extracts to promote health, prevent illness, and support the body's natural healing processes. For thousands of years, herbal remedies have been an integral part of various cultures worldwide, passed down through generations as a treasure trove of traditional knowledge. Today, herbalism continues to thrive, offering a holistic and natural approach to healing.

1.2 Key Terminology

To navigate the world of herbalism, it is essential to familiarize yourself with the terminology commonly used in this field. Let's explore some of the key terms you'll encounter:

a. Infusions: An infusion is made by steeping fresh or dried herbs in hot water. This gentle method extracts the plant's beneficial compounds, resulting in a flavorful herbal tea.

b. Decoctions: Similar to infusions, decoctions involve simmering tougher plant parts, such as roots, bark, or seeds, in water to extract their medicinal properties.

c. Herbal Teas: Herbal teas are an accessible and enjoyable way to consume medicinal plants. They can be made from single herbs or herbal blends, each offering specific health benefits.

d. Ointments: Ointments are topical preparations made by infusing herbs into oils and combining them with beeswax to create a soothing balm for the skin.

e. Tinctures: Tinctures are concentrated liquid extracts of herbs, made by steeping the plant material in alcohol or glycerin to preserve and extract their medicinal constituents.

1.3 Precautions in Herbal Medicine

While herbal medicine can offer valuable health benefits, it is essential to approach it with care and knowledge. Like any form of medicine, medicinal plants can interact with medications or cause allergic reactions in some individuals. Before starting any herbal regimen, consult with a qualified healthcare professional, especially if you are pregnant, breastfeeding, or have underlying health conditions.

1.4 Herbalism's Holistic Approach

Herbalism's strength lies in its holistic approach to health. Rather than solely treating symptoms, herbalists consider the whole person—mind, body, and spirit. By addressing the root causes of imbalances, herbal remedies aim to restore harmony and promote overall well-being.

1.5 Cultivating a Connection with Nature

Herbalism not only offers medicinal benefits but also fosters a deep connection with nature. Growing, harvesting, and preparing medicinal plants can be a profoundly grounding and fulfilling experience. As you embark on your herbal journey, you will likely find yourself forming a stronger bond with the natural world around you.

In this introductory chapter, we have laid the foundation for your exploration of herbalism. By understanding its fundamental principles, key terminology, precautions, and holistic approach, you are now better equipped to embark on the exciting journey of cultivating and using medicinal plants. As we delve deeper into the world of herbal medicine, we will unlock the secrets of various herbs and their therapeutic properties, empowering you to take charge of your health in a natural and sustainable way.

Medicinal Plants: Nature and Therapeutic Potential

Medicinal plants form the foundation of herbal medicine, offering a wide range of health benefits for humans. In this chapter, we will explore the diversity of medicinal plants, their therapeutic potential, and their history in both traditional and modern use. It will be an exciting journey into the world of herbs, where you will discover how these wonders of nature can support your health and well-being in remarkable ways.

2.1 From Nature to Pharmacy

Medicinal plants have been used since ancient times to treat illnesses and disorders and are considered nature's original pharmacy. In various cultures, herbalists have developed a vast treasure trove of knowledge regarding the healing properties of plants, passing down such secrets from generation to generation. Today, with the resurgence of interest in natural therapies, medicinal plants continue to play an essential role in the health and well-being of people worldwide.

2.2 Diversity of Medicinal Plants

Medicinal plants encompass a wide range of botanical species, each with its unique characteristics and therapeutic properties. Some herbs are renowned for their calming effect on the nervous system, while others may help strengthen the immune system or promote wound healing. Let's explore some of the most common categories of medicinal plants:

a. Adaptogens: These plants support the body's adaptation to stress, helping to balance the endocrine system and promoting mental and physical equilibrium.

b. Anti-inflammatories: Plants with anti-inflammatory properties help reduce inflammation and pain in the body, facilitating the healing process.

c. Tonics: Tonic plants strengthen and invigorate the body, increasing physical and mental resilience.

d. Antioxidants: These herbs protect the body from damage caused by free radicals and may help prevent chronic diseases.

e. Sedatives: Sedative plants have a calming effect on the nervous system, helping to reduce anxiety and promote restful sleep.

2.3 Identifying and Harvesting Medicinal Plants

Accurate identification of medicinal plants is crucial to ensure their safety and efficacy. Before harvesting any herb, it is essential to become familiar with its distinctive features, such as leaves, flowers, fruits, and aromas. Misidentification could lead to the use of a toxic or even lethal plant.

2.4 Preparing Medicinal Plants

After harvesting the plants, they need proper preparation to obtain their therapeutic benefits. Preparation methods vary depending on the part of the plant used and the desired form of preparation. Some common methods include:

a. Infusion: Making a herbal tea using soft parts of the plants, such as leaves or flowers, with hot water.

b. Decoction: Boiling tougher parts of the plant, such as roots, barks, or seeds, to extract the active compounds.

c. Tincture: Extracting medicinal compounds using alcohol or glycerine as a solvent.

d. Ointments and Balms: Preparing soothing balms and ointments with oils and medicinal plants for topical use.

2.5 Safety and Contraindications

While medicinal plants offer numerous benefits, it is essential to use them wisely and with care. Some herbs may interact with medications, be contraindicated in certain medical conditions, or cause allergic reactions. Before using any herbal remedy, consult with a qualified professional and educate yourself about any precautions or contraindications.

The world of medicinal plants is vast and fascinating, offering an incredible variety of health benefits. In this chapter, we have explored the diversity of medicinal plants, their history, and their therapeutic potential. By gaining a solid understanding of these aspects, you will be better prepared to use medicinal plants safely and effectively to enhance your health and overall well-being.

Chapter 2: The Therapeutic Power of Herbal Medicine

Herbal medicine has been used for centuries to promote health and alleviate various health conditions. In this chapter, we will delve into the therapeutic power of herbal remedies, exploring how different herbs interact with the body to support healing and well-being. Understanding the mechanisms behind herbal medicine will provide valuable insights into their efficacy and application in modern healthcare practices.

3.1 Active Compounds in Medicinal Plants

Medicinal plants contain a myriad of active compounds, each contributing to their unique therapeutic effects. These bioactive compounds may include alkaloids, flavonoids, terpenoids, phenolic acids, and many others. Understanding the specific compounds present in each herb is essential for tailoring treatments and achieving desired health outcomes.

3.2 Mechanisms of Action

Herbal medicine exerts its effects through various mechanisms of action, often targeting multiple pathways in the body. Some common mechanisms include:

a. Modulating Enzymes: Certain herbs can enhance or inhibit specific enzymes, regulating biochemical processes in the body.

b. Interacting with Receptors: Herbal compounds can bind to receptors in the body, mimicking or blocking the effects of certain hormones or neurotransmitters.

c. Anti-Microbial Properties: Many herbs possess antimicrobial properties, making them effective against bacteria, viruses, and fungi.

d. Anti-Inflammatory Effects: Herbal remedies can help reduce inflammation by inhibiting pro-inflammatory enzymes.

e. Antioxidant Activity: The antioxidant compounds in herbs protect the body's cells from oxidative stress, contributing to overall health.

3.3 Synergy and Holistic Healing

The combination of multiple active compounds in medicinal plants often leads to a phenomenon called synergy. Synergy occurs when the collective action of these compounds enhances the overall therapeutic effect beyond what individual compounds can achieve alone. This holistic approach to healing acknowledges the intricate interplay of plant components and their ability to work in harmony with the body's natural processes.

3.4 Herbal Formulations and Combinations

Herbalists often create formulations that combine different herbs to target specific health issues comprehensively. These synergistic blends aim to address various aspects of a condition, optimizing the chances of successful treatment. Understanding the art of herbal formulations is a valuable skill for herbal practitioners seeking to customize treatments for individual patients.

3.5 Evidence-Based Herbal Medicine

The field of herbal medicine is continually evolving, with ongoing research providing valuable insights into the efficacy and safety of various herbs. Evidence-based herbal medicine relies on scientific studies and clinical trials to support the use of specific herbs for certain health conditions. Integrating evidence-based practices with traditional knowledge ensures a well-rounded and reliable approach to herbal medicine.

3.6 Integrating Herbal Medicine with Conventional Healthcare

As interest in natural remedies grows, the integration of herbal medicine with conventional healthcare becomes increasingly important. Collaboration between herbalists and healthcare professionals fosters a more comprehensive approach to patient care. Understanding the potential interactions between herbal remedies and conventional medications is essential to ensure patient safety and effective treatment outcomes.

In this chapter, we have explored the therapeutic power of herbal medicine, understanding the active compounds, mechanisms of action, and the importance of synergy in achieving holistic healing. By blending traditional knowledge with evidence-based practices and integrating herbal medicine with conventional healthcare, we can harness the full potential of medicinal plants to promote health and well-being effectively.

Herbal Medicine

Herbal medicine is defined as "the knowledge, skills, and methods based on the philosophies, beliefs, and relationships unique to many nations, applied in the health preservation and health prevention, assessment, augmentation, or treatment of the mental and physical problem" Traditional medicine has several various structures. The environment governs each action and theory, particular circumstances, and geographic region in which it originated. Regardless of the underlying condition or sickness the patient has, the focus is often on their overall health, and using herbs is a key component of many traditional medicine regimens.

Traditional Chinese medicine has been a key example of how classical and acquired knowledge is used via a methodical approach to modern medical treatment (TCM). TCM has a more than 3,000-year history. The Devine Farmer's Classic of Herbalism, the world's oldest known herbal treatise, was written in China around 2000 years ago. However, the scientifically documented and accumulated herbal information has developed into multiple herbal pharmacopeias and countless monographs on specific plants.

Treatment and diagnosis are based on a balanced understanding of the illness and its repercussions, as symbolized by the Yin-Yang combination. In contrast to Yang, who represents the sky, masculinity, and heat, yin represents femininity, the soil, and ice. The interactions between the five elements that make up the world—wood, water, metal, earth, and fire— are influenced by yin and Yang. The 12 meridians that TCM practitioners control transport and direct energy (Qi) through a body to varying degrees of Yang and yin. TCM is a growing practice used to promote health and ward off and prevent sickness. TCM involves various activities, although traditional treatments and organic components are key.

The development and mass production of chemically produced medications throughout the last century has changed healthcare in several parts of the world. However, in wealthy nations, sizable portions of the populace also rely on traditional doctors and herbal treatments as the main form of therapy. For their medical requirements, up to 90% of people in Africa and 70% of people in India use conventional medicine. Over 90% of state hospitals in China include traditional medicine departments, and conventional medicine makes up about 40% of all healthcare services offered. However, herbal treatments are not only practiced in developing countries. During the last 20 years, ethnobotanicals have greatly increased the public interest in herbal remedies in industrialized nations.

The most common reasons for using natural remedies are that they are more widely available, more closely align with the patient's lifestyle, allay fears about the negative effects of synthetic (artificial) drugs, satisfy the need for more individualized healthcare, and enable a more thorough community approach to health records. The major uses of herbal medicines are to improve human health, treat chronic illnesses, and prevent serious illnesses. However, as contemporary infectious illnesses and advanced malignancies are managed clinically, natural therapies are becoming increasingly popular. Natural medicines, in contrast, are widely acknowledged, non-toxic, and beneficial.

Herbal medicine is a vital component of health care, whether a person needs it or not, whether they have access to allopathic treatment physically or financially. Its global market is expanding.

Currently, herbs are used to treat various conditions, including heart disease, obesity, asthma, anxiety, and prostate diseases, as well as chronic and severe illnesses, disorders, and concerns. In China in 2003, the strategy for containing and treating SARS (severe acute respiratory syndrome) relied heavily on conventional natural therapies. The African flower is a traditional herbal remedy that has been used for a very long time in Africa to treat HIV-related illnesses. In Europe, natural remedies are still popular. It is common to find herbal extracts, teas, and essential oils at pharmacies that offer prescription pharmaceuticals in most industrialized nations, with France and Germany topping total European purchasing.

Herbs and seeds may be produced and consumed in various forms, including entire herbs, teas, syrups, lavender oil, ointments, salves, rubbers, pills, and capsules containing a powdered dry extract of a raw herb form. In addition to vinegar (extracts of acetic acid), alcoholic extracts, hot water extracts (tisanes), extended boiling extracts, often bark and roots (decoctions), and cold plant infusions, there are other types of plant and herb extracts. There isn't much detail, and the components in herbal products often vary greatly across batches and producers.

There are many different plant species, and their compounds are diverse. The majority are secondary plant metabolites that include aromatic compounds, the majority of which are phenols or phenolic compounds that have had oxygen added, such as tannins. They include a lot of antioxidants.

Cultivation and Harvesting of Medicinal Plants

In the previous chapter, we explored the therapeutic power of medicinal plants. Now, it's time to delve into how to cultivate and harvest these valuable herbs in your garden. Cultivating medicinal plants provides a unique opportunity to develop a deeper connection with nature and obtain high-quality herbs for your personal herbal medicine. In this chapter, we will guide you step by step through the process of preparing the soil, planting, caring for the plants, and harvesting the herbs at the right time to maximize their therapeutic benefits.

4.1 Soil Preparation

Before planting your medicinal herbs, it is crucial to properly prepare the soil to ensure healthy and vigorous growth of the plants. Start by removing weeds and debris from the cultivation area and work the soil with a shovel or fork to loosen it. Be sure to break up any clumps and level the soil surface evenly.

4.2 Selection of Herbal Species and Varieties

When choosing herbs to cultivate, consider your therapeutic needs, local climate, and soil conditions. Opt for herbal species and varieties that are suitable for your climate and environment, so they can thrive with minimal care. Some herbs are perennials, while others are annuals or biennials, so also take into account their lifespan and growth cycle.

4.3 Planting Medicinal Herbs

Once you have chosen the planting location and the herbs to grow, the timing of planting is crucial for the success of your cultivation. Annual herbs can be sown directly into the soil at the beginning of the growing season, while perennial herbs can be planted either through seeds or purchased seedlings from a local nursery. Make sure to follow the recommended planting spacing for each plant to allow for optimal growth.

4.4 Care for Medicinal Plants

Medicinal plants require proper care to thrive and reach their full therapeutic potential. Regularly water the plants, especially during dry periods, but avoid overwatering, which could damage the roots. Prune the herbs to maintain their shape and remove any diseased or damaged parts. Provide support for vertically growing plants to ensure healthy growth.

4.5 Harvesting Medicinal Herbs

Harvesting the herbs at the right time is essential to ensure the highest concentration of active compounds. Each herb has its optimal time for harvesting, which may vary depending on the plant part used (leaves, flowers, roots, etc.). In general, harvest leaves before flowering to obtain the highest content of active constituents. Roots, on the other hand, are best harvested during the autumn rest period when the plant's energy is concentrated in the roots.

4.6 Drying and Storage

After harvesting, properly drying the herbs is essential to preserve their effectiveness and freshness. Lay out the collected plant parts on racks or hang them upside down in a cool, dark, and well-ventilated area. Avoid overcrowding the plants during drying to prevent the formation of mold or mildew. Once dried, store the herbs in sealed containers away from direct sunlight and moisture.

Cultivating and harvesting your medicinal plants is a rewarding experience that allows you to obtain high-quality herbs for your therapeutic needs. By properly preparing the soil, selecting the right herbs, planting them correctly, and caring for the plants, you can harness the healing power of nature to its fullest. Accurate harvesting and drying of the herbs will ensure that your herbal preparations are rich in active compounds and ready to promote your well-being.

Chapter 3: Herbal Medicine Preparations and Applications

In the previous chapters, we explored the art of cultivating and harvesting medicinal plants. Now, let's delve into the various methods of preparing and applying these valuable herbs to harness their healing properties effectively. Herbal medicine preparations come in diverse forms, each tailored to suit specific therapeutic needs. Understanding these preparation methods and their applications is essential for crafting potent remedies for various ailments. In this chapter, we will explore the art of creating herbal infusions, decoctions, tinctures, salves, poultices, and more.

5.1 Herbal Infusions

Herbal infusions, also known as herbal teas, are one of the simplest and most popular methods of extracting medicinal compounds from plants. To make an infusion, pour hot (not boiling) water over the dried or fresh herbs and let them steep for a specified period. Different parts of the plant, such as leaves, flowers, or stems, require varying steeping times to obtain the desired concentration of active constituents. Herbal infusions are typically consumed orally and can provide relief for a range of conditions, including digestive issues, anxiety, and insomnia.

5.2 Herbal Decoctions

Decoctions are similar to infusions, but they involve simmering the plant material in water over low heat for a more extended period. This method is ideal for extracting therapeutic compounds from tougher plant parts like roots, barks, and seeds. Decoctions are often used to address respiratory problems, joint pain, and other ailments that require a higher concentration of active constituents.

5.3 Herbal Tinctures

Herbal tinctures are concentrated liquid extracts made by macerating herbs in alcohol or a mixture of alcohol and water. The alcohol acts as a solvent, drawing out the medicinal compounds from the plant material. Tinctures have a long shelf life and provide a potent and convenient way to administer herbal remedies. They can be taken orally by adding drops to water or other beverages. Additionally, tinctures can be applied topically for localized relief from pain or skin conditions.

5.4 Herbal Salves and Ointments

Salves and ointments are semi-solid herbal preparations that are applied externally to the skin. They are made by infusing herbs in a carrier oil, such as olive or coconut oil, and combining them with beeswax to create a thick consistency. Herbal salves are particularly useful for treating skin conditions, wounds, and muscle aches. When applied topically, they provide a soothing and protective effect.

5.5 Herbal Poultices

Herbal poultices involve applying fresh or dried herbs directly to the affected area. The herbs are often crushed or ground to release their juices and then placed on the skin, covered with a cloth or bandage.

Poultices are valuable for relieving inflammation, bruises, and insect bites. They work by promoting blood circulation and facilitating the penetration of active compounds into the skin.

5.6 Herbal Inhalations

Herbal inhalations, or steam therapies, involve inhaling the steam infused with herbal extracts to address respiratory conditions. To create an herbal inhalation, add dried or fresh herbs to a bowl of hot water, lean over the bowl, and cover your head with a towel to trap the steam. Inhale deeply for several minutes to benefit from the aromatic and therapeutic properties of the herbs.

Mastering the art of herbal medicine preparations opens up a world of possibilities for promoting health and well-being. Whether crafting herbal teas, tinctures, salves, or poultices, each method offers unique therapeutic benefits. By understanding the diverse applications of these herbal preparations, you can create personalized remedies to address a wide array of health concerns. Remember to respect the potency of these natural remedies and seek professional guidance when needed. With dedication and knowledge, you can embark on a fulfilling journey of herbal healing for yourself and others.

Native American Herbalism and Alchemy

Native American herbalism and alchemy represent a rich and profound tradition that has been passed down through generations. These ancient healing practices are deeply connected to nature, spirituality, and the profound understanding of the natural world. In this chapter, we will explore the wisdom of Native American herbalism, which encompasses not only the use of medicinal plants but also a holistic approach to healing that considers the physical, emotional, and spiritual aspects of individuals.

6.1 The Wisdom of Native American Herbalism

Native American herbalism is rooted in a deep reverence for the land and its inhabitants. The indigenous peoples of North America have long understood the healing power of plants and their ability to support the body's natural ability to restore balance and harmony. The knowledge of medicinal plants has been passed down through oral traditions, with each tribe possessing its unique understanding of plant medicine.

6.2 The Role of the Medicine Man and Woman

In Native American communities, medicine men and women, also known as shamans or healers, play a crucial role in the practice of herbalism. These wise individuals possess intimate knowledge of the healing properties of plants and are skilled in using them to address various ailments. They also act as spiritual guides, bridging the gap between the physical and spiritual realms to facilitate healing on multiple levels.

6.3 Sacred Medicinal Plants

Several plants hold sacred significance in Native American herbalism. These plants are revered not only for their healing properties but also for their spiritual and ceremonial uses. Examples of such sacred medicinal plants include sage, cedar, sweetgrass, tobacco, and many others. These plants are often used in purification rituals, prayer ceremonies, and for fostering a connection with the spiritual world.

6.4 The Alchemy of Healing

Native American herbalism goes beyond the physical aspects of healing and embraces the concept of alchemy, where healing is viewed as a transformational process. It involves not only the treatment of symptoms but also a deep exploration of the root causes of illness, which may include emotional and spiritual imbalances. The alchemical approach seeks to restore harmony and alignment with nature and the universe.

6.5 Herbal Rituals and Ceremonies

Herbal rituals and ceremonies are integral to Native American healing practices. These ceremonies often involve the use of medicinal plants, drumming, singing, and dancing to create a sacred and healing space. Rituals may vary among tribes and communities, but they all share the common intention of promoting healing, unity, and connection with the spiritual realm.

6.6 Respecting Traditional Knowledge

As we explore the wisdom of Native American herbalism and alchemy, it is essential to approach this knowledge with deep respect and reverence. Traditional knowledge is a precious legacy that must be preserved and honored. When incorporating Native American healing practices into our lives, it is crucial to do so with humility, cultural sensitivity, and a willingness to learn from the wisdom of the indigenous peoples.

Native American herbalism and alchemy offer profound insights into the interconnectedness of all life and the power of plants to heal and transform. By embracing the wisdom of these ancient traditions, we can cultivate a deeper connection with nature and our own inner healing potential. As we continue on our journey of herbal medicine, let us honor and carry forward the sacred knowledge of Native American healers, integrating their wisdom into our modern approach to holistic healing.

Chapter 4: Essential Oils - Nature's Aromatic Healers

Essential oils have been treasured for their therapeutic properties and captivating fragrances for thousands of years. Derived from aromatic plants, these precious oils carry the essence of nature's healing power. In this chapter, we will delve into the fascinating world of essential oils, exploring their extraction methods, therapeutic uses, and safety considerations. As we unlock the secrets of these aromatic healers, we will discover their potential to support physical, emotional, and spiritual well-being.

7.1 Understanding Essential Oils

Essential oils are highly concentrated plant extracts obtained through various methods, such as steam distillation, cold pressing, or solvent extraction. These potent oils capture the plant's aromatic compounds, which contain the essence and medicinal properties of the plant. Each essential oil boasts a unique chemical composition, giving it distinct therapeutic benefits.

7.2 The Science of Aromatherapy

Aromatherapy is the art and science of using essential oils to enhance overall well-being. When inhaled or applied to the skin, essential oils interact with the body's limbic system, influencing emotions, memory, and mood. Aromatherapy is a complementary healing modality that can be used alongside conventional medicine to promote relaxation, reduce stress, and support emotional balance.

7.3 Popular Essential Oils and Their Uses

There is a vast array of essential oils, each with its own therapeutic properties and applications. We will explore some of the most popular essential oils and their uses:

Lavender (Lavandula angustifolia): Renowned for its calming and soothing properties, lavender is commonly used to promote relaxation, improve sleep quality, and alleviate anxiety.

Peppermint (Mentha piperita): Peppermint essential oil is known for its invigorating and refreshing effects. It can help ease headaches, relieve digestive discomfort, and boost energy levels.

Tea Tree (Melaleuca alternifolia): With powerful antiseptic and antimicrobial properties, tea tree oil is a staple in natural skin care remedies. It is beneficial for treating acne, fungal infections, and insect bites.

Eucalyptus (Eucalyptus globulus): This oil is revered for its respiratory benefits. Eucalyptus can alleviate congestion, soothe coughs, and support respiratory health.

Chamomile (Matricaria chamomilla): Chamomile essential oil is prized for its calming effects. It can help ease tension, promote relaxation, and aid in managing stress and insomnia.

Frankincense (Boswellia carterii): A sacred oil in many cultures, frankincense is renowned for its spiritual and meditative properties. It can promote a sense of grounding and connection during meditation and prayer.

7.4 Application Methods and Safety Precautions

When using essential oils, it is essential to apply them safely and appropriately. Different oils require varying dilution ratios, and some may need to be avoided during pregnancy or certain medical conditions. Common application methods include inhalation, topical application, and diffusion. We will provide detailed guidelines on how to use essential oils safely to maximize their benefits and minimize the risk of adverse reactions.

7.5 Blending Essential Oils

Creating custom blends of essential oils allows you to tailor their therapeutic effects to your specific needs and preferences. We will explore the art of blending essential oils, discussing the principles of complementary scents and the science behind creating harmonious blends. Whether you are seeking relaxation, energy, or emotional support, blending essential oils can be a creative and effective way to harness their healing potential.

7.6 Incorporating Aromatherapy into Daily Life

Aromatherapy is a versatile practice that can be easily integrated into daily life. From using essential oils in diffusers to crafting personalized body oils, bath salts, and sprays, we will provide practical tips and recipes to help you incorporate aromatherapy into your self-care routine. Discover how to create a calming bedtime ritual, an energizing morning routine, or a soothing space for meditation.

7.7 The Power of Scent and Memory

Scent has a profound impact on our memories and emotions. We will explore the connection between scent and memory, understanding how certain aromas can evoke past experiences and emotions. By harnessing the power of scent, we can use essential oils to create positive associations and support emotional healing.

Essential oils offer a treasure trove of therapeutic benefits and aromatic delights. From promoting physical healing to supporting emotional well-being, these gifts of nature have the power to enhance our lives on multiple levels. By understanding their unique properties and practicing aromatherapy with care and respect, we can harness the full potential of essential oils and embrace nature's aromatic healers as powerful allies on our journey to holistic wellness.

Herbal Remedies for Common Ailments - Nature's Healing Panacea

In this chapter, we will explore the world of herbal remedies and their time-honored tradition of healing. Herbal medicine has been practiced for centuries, drawing on the wisdom of ancient civilizations and indigenous cultures. From alleviating minor ailments to supporting overall wellness, herbs have been regarded as nature's healing panacea. Join us as we delve into the diverse world of herbal remedies, uncovering their therapeutic uses, preparation methods, and evidence-based benefits.

8.1 Understanding Herbal Medicine

Herbal medicine, also known as herbalism, is the use of plants and plant extracts to promote health and treat various ailments. It is a holistic approach that considers not only the physical symptoms but also the underlying imbalances in the body. Herbal remedies work synergistically with the body's natural healing processes, offering gentle yet potent support.

8.2 The Healing Power of Common Herbs

We will explore a selection of commonly used herbs and their therapeutic properties:

Calendula (Calendula officinalis): Known for its soothing and anti-inflammatory properties, calendula is beneficial for skin irritations, minor cuts, and burns.

Echinacea (Echinacea purpurea): A popular immune-boosting herb, echinacea can help prevent and reduce the severity of colds and flu.

Ginger (Zingiber officinale): With its warming and anti-nausea properties, ginger is an effective remedy for digestive discomfort and motion sickness.

Chamomile (Matricaria chamomilla): Chamomile's gentle calming effects make it a go-to herb for promoting relaxation and relieving stress.

Peppermint (Mentha piperita): Peppermint aids in digestion, eases headaches, and offers a refreshing and cooling sensation.

Valerian (Valeriana officinalis): A natural sedative, valerian can improve sleep quality and reduce insomnia and anxiety.

8.3 Preparing Herbal Remedies

Discover the various methods of preparing herbal remedies, such as teas, infusions, decoctions, tinctures, and herbal oils. Each preparation method extracts different constituents from the plant, making them suitable for different therapeutic purposes. We will provide step-by-step instructions for preparing herbal remedies at home, empowering you to become your own herbalist.

8.4 Evidence-Based Benefits of Herbal Medicine

While herbal remedies have a long history of traditional use, modern scientific research has also shed light on their therapeutic benefits. We will delve into the evidence-based benefits of specific herbs and explore how they can complement conventional medicine. From supporting cardiovascular health to managing stress and anxiety, we will highlight the growing body of research supporting the efficacy of herbal medicine.

8.5 Integrating Herbal Medicine with Conventional Care

Herbal medicine can be a valuable addition to conventional medical treatments. We will discuss how to integrate herbal remedies safely and effectively with conventional care, ensuring they enhance each other's benefits while avoiding potential interactions. Consultation with healthcare professionals is essential, especially when addressing chronic or severe health conditions.

8.6 Herbal Remedies for the Whole Family

Herbal medicine is suitable for individuals of all ages, from infants to the elderly. We will explore age-appropriate herbal remedies for common ailments, ensuring that the whole family can benefit from nature's healing gifts. Safety considerations and proper dosages for children and seniors will be discussed to ensure their well-being.

8.7 Growing and Cultivating Medicinal Herbs

For those with green thumbs and a passion for gardening, we will provide guidance on growing and cultivating medicinal herbs at home. Cultivating your healing garden allows you to have a readily available supply of fresh herbs for your herbal remedies, fostering a deeper connection with nature and the healing process.

Herbal remedies have stood the test of time, offering a holistic and gentle approach to healing. As we continue to explore the therapeutic properties of common herbs and their evidence-based benefits, we are reminded of the wisdom and generosity of natureEmbracing herbal medicine empowers us to take charge of our health and well-being, tapping into the abundance of nature's healing panacea. Whether you seek to alleviate common ailments or support overall wellness, herbal remedies are a timeless ally on your journey to optimal health and vitality.

Chapter 5: A Natural Approach to Children's Health - Nurturing Wellness from the Start

In this chapter, we will explore the world of natural remedies and holistic approaches to children's health. As parents and caregivers, our top priority is to ensure the well-being of our little ones. Natural remedies offer safe and effective solutions to support children's health, from boosting their immune systems to addressing common childhood ailments. Join us as we delve into the gentle and nurturing world of herbal medicine for children.

9.1 The Foundations of Children's Health

The well-being of children starts with a strong foundation. We will discuss the importance of nutrition, sleep, and emotional well-being in supporting children's overall health. A balanced diet rich in nutrients, restful sleep, and a nurturing environment play vital roles in fostering their physical, emotional, and mental development.

9.2 Herbal Remedies for Common Childhood Ailments

Children are susceptible to various common ailments, such as colds, coughs, fevers, and digestive issues. We will explore a range of gentle herbal remedies to address these concerns. From soothing chamomile tea for restful sleep to elderberry syrup for boosting their immune system, these natural remedies can provide comfort and relief for your little ones.

9.3 Building a Natural First Aid Kit

Accidents and minor injuries are a part of childhood. We will guide you in creating a natural first aid kit, equipped with herbal salves, balms, and tinctures to address cuts, bruises, and skin irritations. Natural first aid empowers you to respond quickly and effectively to your child's needs while avoiding the use of harsh chemicals.

9.4 Supporting Emotional Well-being

Emotional well-being is an integral part of children's health. We will explore herbal remedies that can help alleviate stress, anxiety, and restlessness in children. From calming lavender aromatherapy to gentle herbal teas, these remedies create a soothing and nurturing environment for emotional balance.

9.5 Integrating Natural Remedies with Pediatric Care

Consultation with pediatric healthcare professionals is crucial when using natural remedies for children. We will discuss how to work collaboratively with pediatricians to integrate natural remedies with conventional care. Communication and understanding between caregivers and healthcare providers ensure a holistic and safe approach to children's health.

9.6 Herbal Precautions and Dosages for Children

While natural remedies are generally safe for children, there are specific precautions and dosages to consider based on age and weight. We will provide guidelines and safety considerations to ensure the proper use of herbal remedies for children, empowering you to make informed decisions about their health.

9.7 Nurturing Nature's Connection

Introducing children to the wonders of nature fosters a lifelong appreciation for the environment and its healing gifts. We will discuss nature-based activities and herbal explorations that encourage children to connect with the natural world. These experiences instill a sense of wonder, curiosity, and respect for the healing power of plants.

Nurturing children's health with natural remedies and a holistic approach is a gift that lasts a lifetime. By embracing the gentle and nurturing world of herbal medicine, we can support our children's well-being from the start. From common childhood ailments to emotional balance, herbal remedies provide safe and effective solutions. As caregivers, we have the opportunity to empower our children with natural tools that nurture their health and strengthen their connection to the world around them. Embrace the gentle power of herbal medicine and watch your little ones thrive in health and happiness.

Native American Wisdom - Herbal Traditions and Alchemy

In this chapter, we will delve into the rich and ancient herbal traditions of Native American cultures. Native American tribes have long relied on the healing power of plants to maintain physical, emotional, and spiritual well-being. Their deep connection to the land and profound respect for nature's gifts have shaped a unique system of herbal medicine. Join us on a journey to discover the wisdom and alchemy of Native American herbalism.

10.1 The Sacred Relationship with Nature

Central to Native American herbalism is the sacred relationship between humans and the natural world. We will explore the spiritual beliefs and practices that underpin their approach to herbal medicine. From ceremonies that honor the plant spirits to the concept of interconnectedness, Native American wisdom offers profound insights into the healing potential of the earth.

10.2 Plant Identification and Harvesting

Accurate plant identification and sustainable harvesting practices are essential in Native American herbalism. We will learn how to recognize and respectfully harvest medicinal plants from the wild, ensuring the preservation of these valuable resources. This knowledge is passed down through generations, emphasizing the importance of ecological balance and responsible stewardship of the land.

10.3 Traditional Healing Techniques

Native American herbalism encompasses a wide array of traditional healing techniques. We will explore time-honored methods such as making herbal infusions, decoctions, and poultices. Additionally, we will discuss the significance of smudging and herbal baths as purification rituals, promoting both physical and spiritual cleansing.

10.4 Medicinal Plants and Their Uses

The Native American herbal repertoire includes a diverse range of medicinal plants with specific therapeutic properties. We will study the uses of well-known plants like echinacea, yarrow, and sage, as well as lesser-known gems like bearberry and red root. Understanding the properties and applications of these plants allows us to tap into the richness of Native American herbalism.

10.5 Plant Spirit Medicine

In Native American herbalism, the healing power of plants is believed to be enhanced by connecting with the spirit of the plant. We will explore the concept of plant spirit medicine and its significance in the healing process. Through reverence and intention, Native American healers tap into the spiritual essence of plants to facilitate profound healing.

10.6 Honoring Ancestral Wisdom

The transmission of herbal knowledge in Native American tribes is deeply rooted in ancestral traditions. We will honor the wisdom passed down through generations and acknowledge the importance of preserving and respecting these sacred teachings. Understanding the lineage of herbal knowledge enhances our appreciation for the holistic approach of Native American healing practices.

10.7 Alchemical Practices and Rituals

Alchemy is an integral aspect of Native American herbalism, transforming plants into potent remedies through sacred rituals. We will explore alchemical practices such as fermentation, extraction, and blending, which enhance the medicinal properties of herbal preparations. Embracing the alchemical nature of herbal medicine deepens our connection to the plants and their healing potential.

10.8 Modern Applications of Native American Herbalism

In the modern world, Native American herbalism continues to find relevance and significance. We will discuss how traditional herbal knowledge adapts to contemporary times, integrating with conventional medicine and holistic practices. The bridging of ancient wisdom with modern applications empowers individuals to embrace a holistic approach to wellness.

Native American herbalism offers a profound tapestry of wisdom, reverence, and alchemy that honors the healing gifts of the earth. Through their sacred relationship with nature and deep understanding of plants, Native American cultures have preserved a treasure trove of herbal knowledge. By embracing the principles of this ancient tradition, we gain insight into our interconnectedness with the natural world and the healing potential it holds. Let us honor the wisdom of Native American herbalism and continue to weave the threads of ancestral knowledge into the fabric of our modern lives.

Chapter 6: A Natural Approach to Common Ailments

In this chapter, we will explore the power of herbal remedies in addressing common ailments that affect our daily lives. Embracing a natural approach to wellness allows us to harness the healing properties of plants to support our body's innate ability to heal. Let us delve into the world of herbal solutions for everyday health challenges, providing gentle and effective alternatives to conventional medicine.

11.1 Herbal Support for Digestive Health

The digestive system plays a crucial role in overall well-being, and herbal remedies can offer relief from common digestive issues. We will discuss the use of soothing herbs like peppermint and chamomile for easing indigestion and bloating. Additionally, we will explore herbs that promote healthy gut flora and support optimal digestive function.

11.2 Nurturing the Immune System

A robust immune system is essential for protecting our bodies from illness. We will explore immune-boosting herbs like echinacea, astragalus, and elderberry, which have been used for centuries to fortify the body's defenses against infections and viruses. Understanding how to bolster our immune system naturally empowers us to stay resilient and vibrant.

11.3 Calming the Mind and Easing Stress

In our fast-paced modern world, stress and anxiety have become common challenges. Herbal medicine offers an array of calming herbs like lavender, passionflower, and lemon balm to soothe the mind and promote relaxation. We will explore how these natural remedies can help manage stress and foster emotional well-being.

11.4 Supporting Healthy Sleep

Quality sleep is vital for overall health and vitality. We will discuss herbs such as valerian, chamomile, and skullcap, renowned for their sedative properties and ability to promote restful sleep. Discovering herbal sleep remedies allows us to embrace restorative rest without the need for pharmaceutical sleep aids.

11.5 Herbal Solutions for Respiratory Health

The respiratory system can face various challenges, from seasonal allergies to congestion and coughs. We will explore the use of herbs like mullein, thyme, and eucalyptus, which have long been used to support respiratory health. Understanding how these herbs work synergistically with the body empowers us to navigate respiratory discomfort naturally.

11.6 Herbal Remedies for Skin Care

Our skin is our body's largest organ, and herbal remedies can enhance its health and radiance. We will explore the uses of herbs like calendula, aloe vera, and tea tree oil in soothing skin irritations, promoting skin rejuvenation, and supporting overall skin health.

11.7 Herbs for Women's Health

Herbal medicine offers valuable support for women's health at various stages of life. We will discuss herbs like red raspberry leaf for menstrual health, black cohosh for menopause symptoms, and chasteberry for hormonal balance. Embracing herbal remedies for women's health fosters a deeper connection to the natural rhythms of the body.

11.8 Natural Relief for Muscular Discomfort

Muscular discomfort and tension are common complaints that can be addressed with herbal remedies. We will explore herbs like arnica, cayenne, and ginger, which have analgesic and anti-inflammatory properties to ease muscle soreness and promote flexibility.

11.9 Herbal Care for Children and Families

Herbal remedies are gentle and safe options for supporting the health of children and families. We will discuss child-friendly herbs like chamomile for soothing teething discomfort, elderberry for immune support, and catnip for promoting relaxation. Learning how to integrate herbal care into family wellness empowers parents to take a natural and nurturing approach to health.

A natural approach to common ailments allows us to harness the healing power of plants and embrace the wisdom of herbal remedies. From digestive health to immune support, stress relief to skin care, and beyond, herbs offer a gentle and effective way to nurture our well-being. As we delve into the world of herbal solutions, we are reminded of nature's abundant gifts and the profound impact they can have on our health and vitality. Let us continue to explore the bountiful realm of herbal medicine and integrate these natural remedies into our daily lives for optimal well-being.

How to Become an Expert Herbalist

Becoming an expert herbalist is a rewarding journey that requires dedication, knowledge, and hands-on experience. In this chapter, we will delve into the essential steps to embark on this path and develop a profound understanding of herbal medicine. Whether you are a beginner or already have some herbal knowledge, this chapter will guide you in honing your skills and deepening your connection with the plant world.

12.1 Embrace the Foundations of Herbalism

To become an expert herbalist, it is crucial to start with a solid foundation. We will explore the principles of herbal medicine, understanding the concept of holistic healing, the energetics of plants, and the importance of sustainability and ethical harvesting. By grounding ourselves in these fundamental aspects, we set the stage for a meaningful and effective herbal practice.

12.2 Dive into Botany and Plant Identification

A vital aspect of herbalism is knowing the plants we work with intimately. We will delve into botany, learning about plant families, morphology, and characteristics that aid in plant identification. Understanding how to differentiate between look-alike plants and recognizing them in their natural habitats are essential skills for any herbalist.

12.3 Study Herbal Actions and Constituents

Herbs exert their effects through various actions and constituents. We will explore herbal actions like diuretic, nervine, and astringent, as well as the active compounds responsible for these actions. By understanding how herbs interact with the body, we can effectively choose the right herbs for specific health conditions.

12.4 Create a Home Herbal Apothecary

A well-stocked herbal apothecary is a herbalist's treasure trove. We will discuss how to create a diverse collection of dried herbs, tinctures, oils, and essential oils to address a wide range of health concerns. Building a comprehensive home apothecary allows us to be prepared to support ourselves and others on their wellness journey.

12.5 Master the Art of Herbal Preparations

Herbal preparations are the tools through which we extract and utilize the healing properties of plants. We will explore various methods like infusions, decoctions, tinctures, salves, and herbal syrups, and learn when to use each preparation for maximum efficacy. Mastering the art of herbal preparations empowers us to customize remedies based on individual needs.

12.6 Cultivate Wildcrafting and Growing Herbs

Wildcrafting and growing herbs are essential skills for every herbalist. We will discuss sustainable wildcrafting practices, including ethical harvesting and conserving wild plant populations. Additionally, we will explore how to cultivate a herbal garden, providing us with a readily available supply of fresh herbs to use in our preparations.

12.7 Understand Herbal Safety and Contraindications

Safety is paramount in herbal practice. We will explore the potential side effects and contraindications of herbs, as well as herb-drug interactions to ensure the responsible use of herbal remedies. Understanding herbal safety allows us to provide the best care for ourselves and those seeking our expertise.

12.8 Develop Clinical Skills and Case Studies

To become an expert herbalist, gaining clinical experience is invaluable. We will discuss how to work with clients, take comprehensive health histories, and develop personalized herbal protocols. Real-life case studies will aid in honing our diagnostic skills and understanding the intricacies of individual health journeys.

12.9 Continue Learning and Stay Curious

Herbalism is a lifelong journey of learning and discovery. We will explore resources for continuing education, including books, courses, workshops, and networking with other herbalists. Staying curious and open to new information ensures that we grow and evolve as herbal practitioners.

Becoming an expert herbalist is a profound and transformative journey. By embracing the foundations of herbalism, developing plant identification skills, mastering herbal preparations, and cultivating a connection with nature, we step into the role of a steward of the plant world. As we deepen our knowledge, practice ethical and sustainable herbalism, and continue to learn and grow, we can confidently offer our expertise to support others on their path to wellness. May this chapter inspire you to embark on the rich and fulfilling path of becoming an expert herbalist.

Chapter 7: Herbalism for a Sustainable Future

In this final chapter, we explore the vital role of herbalism in promoting a sustainable and harmonious future for both humanity and the planet. As herbalists, we have a unique opportunity to cultivate a deep connection with nature and advocate for practices that honor and preserve the delicate balance of the natural world. Let us delve into the ways in which herbalism can contribute to a more sustainable future.

13.1 Understanding Ecological Impact

As herbalists, it is essential to understand the ecological impact of our practices. We will explore the concept of bioregional herbalism, focusing on utilizing native plants and supporting local ecosystems. By appreciating the delicate interplay between plants, wildlife, and the environment, we can make conscious choices to minimize our ecological footprint.

13.2 Embracing Ethical Wildcrafting

Ethical wildcrafting is at the core of sustainable herbalism. We will discuss the principles of ethical harvesting, such as gathering in small quantities, respecting plant populations, and obtaining proper permissions when harvesting from private or protected lands. By treading lightly on the earth and ensuring the longevity of wild plant species, we contribute to the preservation of biodiversity.

13.3 Cultivating Medicinal Gardens

Growing our medicinal herbs allows us to be self-sufficient and reduces our dependence on wild harvesting. We will delve into the art of cultivating medicinal gardens, selecting appropriate plants, and creating nurturing environments for their growth. Medicinal gardens not only provide us with a sustainable source of herbs but also become sanctuaries for biodiversity and beneficial insects.

13.4 Supporting Organic and Regenerative Agriculture

As herbalists, we can champion organic and regenerative agricultural practices. We will explore the benefits of supporting local farmers who use organic methods and regenerative techniques to enhance soil health and minimize environmental impact. By endorsing sustainable agriculture, we contribute to healthier ecosystems and cleaner, more potent herbal products.

13.5 Promoting Herbal Education and Community Engagement

Education is a powerful tool for promoting sustainable practices. We will discuss the importance of sharing herbal knowledge with communities and fostering a culture of sustainability. Engaging in community projects, workshops, and educational events allows us to inspire others to connect with nature and embrace herbal remedies as a sustainable form of healing.

13.6 Advocating for Conservation Efforts

Herbalists can play a vital role in advocating for the conservation of endangered plant species and protected habitats. We will explore the importance of supporting conservation organizations and participating in initiatives that focus on preserving at-risk plants. Our collective efforts can make a significant impact in safeguarding the plant diversity essential for future generations.

13.7 Embracing Zero-Waste Herbalism

Minimizing waste in herbal practices is essential for sustainability. We will discuss techniques for zero-waste herbalism, such as making the most of plant materials, composting herbal waste, and using eco-friendly packaging. By adopting zero-waste principles, we demonstrate our commitment to environmental stewardship.

As we conclude our journey through herbalism, let us remember that our actions as herbalists have a profound impact on the world around us. By embracing sustainable practices, supporting biodiversity, and advocating for a harmonious relationship with nature, we contribute to building a more resilient and sustainable future. Herbalism is not merely a collection of remedies; it is a way of life that celebrates our deep connection with the natural world. May our collective efforts as herbalists inspire positive change and foster a thriving and sustainable future for all beings on Earth.

Integrating Herbalism with Modern Medicine

In recent years, there has been a growing interest in integrating traditional herbal medicine with modern healthcare practices. This chapter delves into the potential benefits and challenges of combining herbalism with conventional medicine. While each approach has its strengths, collaboration between herbalists and healthcare professionals can offer comprehensive care and better outcomes for patients.

The Complementary Nature of Herbal Medicine and Modern Healthcare:

Herbal medicine and modern medicine each have unique strengths. Herbalism emphasizes a holistic approach to healing, taking into account the interconnectedness of the body, mind, and spirit. Modern medicine, on the other hand, excels in acute care, surgical interventions, and advanced diagnostics. By combining both approaches, patients can experience a more comprehensive and balanced form of healthcare.

Herbs as Adjuncts to Conventional Treatments:

Herbs can be valuable adjuncts to conventional treatments. In certain cases, herbs may help mitigate side effects of medications or support the body's natural healing processes during recovery. We'll explore specific examples where herbal remedies have been used alongside conventional treatments to enhance patient outcomes.

The Importance of Evidence-Based Herbal Medicine:

Integrating herbalism with modern medicine demands a commitment to evidence-based practices. We'll discuss the significance of research and clinical studies to establish the safety and efficacy of herbal treatments.

Integrative healthcare settings can benefit from combining scientific knowledge with traditional wisdom to optimize patient care.

Collaborating with Healthcare Professionals:

Building effective collaborations between herbalists and healthcare professionals is vital for successful integrative care. We'll provide guidance on communication and sharing information to ensure seamless patient management. By working together, practitioners can create personalized treatment plans that address patients' unique needs.

Navigating Herb-Drug Interactions:

Understanding potential interactions between herbs and pharmaceutical drugs is crucial for patient safety. We'll discuss the importance of a thorough patient history to identify contraindications and herb-drug interactions. This knowledge allows healthcare providers to tailor treatment plans and avoid adverse effects.

Integrative Case Studies:

In this section, we'll explore real-life case studies where patients have benefitted from the integration of herbal medicine with modern treatments. These examples highlight the power of an integrative approach in addressing complex health conditions.

Education and Advocacy for Integrative Care:

To promote the integration of herbalism and modern medicine, education and advocacy are essential. We'll discuss how herbalists can collaborate with healthcare organizations, contribute to research initiatives, and participate in interprofessional training programs.

The Future of Integrative Healthcare:

As the healthcare landscape continues to evolve, integrative medicine is gaining recognition and support. We'll explore the potential growth of integrative healthcare practices and how herbal medicine can play a significant role in the future of patient-centered care.

Integrating herbalism with modern medicine presents a unique opportunity to provide comprehensive and patient-centered care. By fostering collaborations, emphasizing evidence-based practices, and respecting each approach's strengths, we can create a healthcare system that combines the best of both worlds and enhances overall well-being for individuals and communities.

Chapter 8: Sustainable Herbalism and Conservation

As herbalism gains popularity, it is essential to address the importance of sustainable practices and conservation efforts. In this chapter, we will explore the principles of sustainable herbalism and how herbalists can contribute to preserving and protecting our natural resources for future generations.

Understanding Sustainable Herbalism:

Sustainable herbalism involves the responsible use of medicinal plants while ensuring their long-term viability in their natural habitats. We'll discuss the principles of sustainability, including ethical wildcrafting, cultivation, and the importance of preserving biodiversity.

Ethical Wildcrafting and Harvesting:

Wildcrafting, the practice of gathering herbs from their natural environment, requires ethical considerations. We'll delve into guidelines for sustainable wildcrafting, such as harvesting in moderation, respecting plant populations, and choosing ethical suppliers.

Cultivating Medicinal Plants:

Growing medicinal plants in a sustainable manner can alleviate pressure on wild populations. We'll explore the basics of herbal gardening, including selecting appropriate plants, organic cultivation methods, and the benefits of growing native species.

Conservation and Habitat Preservation:

Preserving the habitats of medicinal plants is vital for their survival. We'll discuss the importance of conservation efforts, such as supporting protected areas, engaging in habitat restoration, and advocating for sustainable land use practices.

Endangered and At-Risk Medicinal Plants:

Several medicinal plant species are endangered or at risk due to overharvesting and habitat destruction. We'll highlight some of these vulnerable plants and discuss initiatives to protect and preserve them.

Regulatory Considerations for Sustainable Herbalism:

In many regions, herbalists must navigate regulations and laws concerning the harvesting and trade of medicinal plants. We'll provide an overview of regulatory considerations and how herbalists can stay compliant with local and international laws.

Collaborating with Conservation Organizations:

Herbalists can make a significant impact by collaborating with conservation organizations and supporting their initiatives. We'll explore ways to get involved, support conservation efforts, and raise awareness about the importance of preserving medicinal plant species.

Sustainable Sourcing for Herbal Products:

Consumers play a crucial role in promoting sustainable herbalism by choosing products from ethical and eco-friendly sources. We'll discuss how to identify products that align with sustainability values and the importance of supporting companies committed to responsible sourcing.

Educating the Herbal Community and Public:

Education is a key component of promoting sustainable herbalism. We'll explore ways to educate fellow herbalists, healthcare practitioners, and the public about sustainable practices, conservation, and the importance of protecting our natural resources.

Herbalism and Environmental Stewardship:

Herbalists have a unique opportunity to be environmental stewards, caring for the Earth while promoting health and well-being. We'll discuss how herbalism can be a force for positive change in preserving the environment.

Sustainable herbalism and conservation efforts are essential to ensure the continued availability of medicinal plants for generations to come. By adopting ethical practices, supporting conservation initiatives, and advocating for sustainable policies, herbalists can play a vital role in protecting our natural heritage and fostering a healthier planet.

Herbal First Aid and Emergency Preparedness

In times of emergencies and unexpected situations, herbal first aid can be a valuable skill to have. This chapter will focus on building a comprehensive herbal first aid kit and understanding the essential herbs and remedies that can address common injuries and health issues in emergency situations.

Building Your Herbal First Aid Kit:

We'll begin by discussing the components of a well-rounded herbal first aid kit. From basic supplies like bandages and scissors to essential herbal remedies, we'll guide you through assembling a practical and portable kit for use at home or on the go.

Herbs for Wound Care:

In this section, we'll explore various herbs renowned for their wound-healing properties. From calendula and comfrey to yarrow and plantain, you'll learn how to use these herbs to clean wounds, promote tissue regeneration, and prevent infections.

Herbs for Pain Relief:

Pain can be a common occurrence in emergencies, and knowing which herbs can provide relief is valuable. We'll delve into analgesic herbs such as willow bark, meadowsweet, and Jamaican dogwood, discussing their benefits and administration methods.

Herbs for Digestive Distress:

During emergency situations, digestive issues can arise due to stress or changes in diet. We'll discuss herbal remedies to address common digestive problems, including upset stomach, diarrhea, and nausea.

Herbs for Respiratory Support:

Respiratory issues can become a concern in certain emergencies. We'll explore herbs that can provide respiratory support, like mullein, thyme, and elecampane, and discuss methods of administration for maximum effectiveness.

Herbal Remedies for Anxiety and Stress:

In high-stress situations, herbal remedies can offer calming and soothing effects. We'll discuss herbs like chamomile, lemon balm, and passionflower that can help alleviate anxiety and promote relaxation.

Herbs for Immune Support:

Maintaining a strong immune system is crucial in emergencies. We'll highlight immune-boosting herbs such as echinacea, elderberry, and astragalus, and explore ways to incorporate them into your first aid regimen.

Herbs for Allergic Reactions:

Allergic reactions can occur unexpectedly, and it's essential to be prepared. We'll discuss herbs like nettle, quercetin, and licorice that can help manage mild allergic reactions.

Herbal Remedies for Burns and Sunburns:

Burns are common injuries, especially during emergencies or outdoor activities. We'll cover herbs like aloe vera, lavender, and chamomile that can provide relief and support healing for minor burns and sunburns.

Herbal First Aid for Insect Bites and Stings:

Insect bites and stings can cause discomfort and allergic reactions. We'll explore herbs like plantain, witch hazel, and basil that can soothe insect bites and alleviate itching and inflammation.

Using Herbal First Aid in Different Scenarios:

This section will cover practical applications of herbal first aid in various emergency scenarios, such as natural disasters, outdoor activities, and travel situations.

Having a well-prepared herbal first aid kit and knowledge of effective herbal remedies can make a significant difference in emergency situations. By incorporating herbal first aid into your preparedness plan, you can be better equipped to handle unexpected health issues and injuries with natural and effective solutions.

Chapter 9: Integrating Herbal Medicine into Everyday Life

As you've learned about the various aspects of herbal medicine, it's essential to understand how to integrate these practices into your daily life. This chapter will focus on incorporating herbal remedies and practices seamlessly into your lifestyle to promote overall well-being and improve health.

Creating Herbal Rituals:

Herbal rituals can be a meaningful way to connect with nature and the healing properties of plants. We'll explore how to create simple yet powerful herbal rituals, such as morning herbal infusions, evening relaxation teas, and mindful herbal baths, to enhance your daily routines.

Herbal Skincare and Beauty:

Taking care of your skin with herbal-infused products can be a delightful and rejuvenating experience. We'll discuss how to make herbal skincare products like facial serums, body scrubs, and herbal face masks to nourish and revitalize your skin naturally.

Herbal Hair Care:

Your hair can benefit from herbal care too. We'll explore herbal hair rinses, scalp treatments, and hair oils to promote healthy hair growth, reduce dandruff, and add shine to your locks.

Herbs for Stress Management:

Stress is a common part of modern life, and herbal remedies can play a significant role in managing it. We'll discuss adaptogenic herbs like ashwagandha, holy basil, and rhodiola, which can help the body adapt to stress and restore balance.

Herbal Sleep Support:

Quality sleep is vital for overall well-being. We'll explore calming herbs such as valerian, passionflower, and California poppy, and techniques like creating a bedtime herbal routine to promote restful and rejuvenating sleep.

Herbal Nutrition and Culinary Delights:

Enhancing your culinary skills with herbal ingredients can elevate the nutritional value and flavors of your meals. We'll discuss how to incorporate herbs into cooking, creating herbal oils, herbal vinegar, and herbal-infused salts to add a touch of herbal goodness to your dishes.

Herbs for Emotional Wellness:

Herbs can have a profound impact on emotional health and balance. We'll explore herbs like St. John's Wort, lemon balm, and lavender, which can support emotional well-being and help manage feelings of sadness, anxiety, and irritability.

Herbal Remedies for Common Ailments:

Incorporating herbal remedies into your daily life means having go-to solutions for common ailments. We'll create a handy guide for using herbs to address issues like headaches, indigestion, seasonal allergies, and minor injuries.

Herbal Teas and Tonics:

Herbal teas and tonics can be delightful beverages to enjoy throughout the day. We'll explore different herbal blends and tonics to support specific health needs, from immune-boosting teas to digestive tonics.

Growing and Harvesting Your Own Herbs:

Having your herbal garden is not only rewarding but also ensures a fresh and sustainable supply of herbs. We'll provide tips on growing and harvesting your herbs, including proper drying and storage techniques.

Herbal Medicine for Children and Pets:

Herbal remedies can be safe and effective for children and pets when used correctly. We'll discuss how to adapt herbal medicine for their needs, providing natural solutions for common childhood ailments and pet health issues.

By integrating herbal medicine into your everyday life, you can experience the full benefits of these natural remedies and practices. Whether it's creating herbal rituals, using herbal skincare products, or incorporating herbs into your culinary creations, embracing herbal medicine as a lifestyle choice can lead to a healthier, more balanced, and harmonious way of living. Remember to always seek professional advice when needed and enjoy the journey of exploring the wonderful world of herbal medicine.

The Future of Herbal Medicine

As we conclude this comprehensive journey through herbal medicine, it is essential to consider the future of this ancient healing practice. In this chapter, we will explore the evolving landscape of herbal medicine, including emerging trends, scientific advancements, and the importance of preserving traditional knowledge.

The Resurgence of Herbal Medicine:

Herbal medicine is experiencing a resurgence in popularity as people seek more natural and holistic approaches to health and wellness. We'll discuss the reasons behind this resurgence and how herbal medicine is gaining recognition and acceptance in mainstream healthcare.

Herbal Medicine and Modern Science:

The integration of traditional herbal knowledge with modern scientific research is a promising area of development. We'll delve into current scientific studies that explore the medicinal properties of herbs, validating their traditional uses and discovering new applications.

Sustainable Herbal Practices:

With the growing demand for herbal remedies, it becomes crucial to prioritize sustainability and ethical harvesting. We'll explore sustainable practices for growing, harvesting, and sourcing herbs to protect biodiversity and support the long-term availability of medicinal plants.

Herbal Medicine and Cultural Preservation:

Herbal medicine is deeply rooted in various cultures and indigenous traditions. We'll discuss the significance of preserving and respecting these traditional knowledge systems and the role of herbal medicine in cultural identity.

The Role of Technology in Herbal Medicine:

Advancements in technology are shaping the future of herbal medicine. From herbal databases and smartphone apps that aid in plant identification to innovative extraction methods, we'll explore how technology is enhancing our understanding and use of herbal remedies.

Herbal Medicine Education and Certification:

As interest in herbal medicine grows, the need for well-trained practitioners becomes more significant. We'll discuss the importance of standardized herbal medicine education, certification, and the role of professional herbalists in promoting safe and effective herbal practices.

Herbal Medicine and Global Health:

The accessibility and affordability of herbal medicine make it a valuable resource for global health initiatives. We'll explore how herbal medicine can contribute to improving healthcare in underserved communities and developing regions.

Challenges and Opportunities in Herbal Medicine:

Despite its many benefits, herbal medicine faces challenges, including regulatory issues and misinformation. We'll address these challenges and discuss opportunities for promoting responsible herbal practices and bridging the gap between traditional and modern medicine.

Personalizing Herbal Medicine:

Each individual's health needs are unique, and personalized herbal medicine can provide tailored solutions. We'll explore the concept of individualized herbal protocols and how they can optimize health outcomes.

Herbal Medicine and Mental Health:

The connection between herbal medicine and mental health is gaining recognition. We'll discuss the role of herbs in supporting emotional well-being and their potential as complementary therapies for mental health conditions.

The Holistic Approach of Herbal Medicine:

Herbal medicine embraces a holistic approach that considers the interconnectedness of the mind, body, and spirit. We'll explore how this holistic perspective can lead to a deeper understanding of health and healing.

The future of herbal medicine is filled with promise and potential. As we continue to integrate traditional wisdom with modern science and technology, herbal medicine's role in promoting health and wellness will undoubtedly expand. By embracing sustainability, preserving cultural knowledge, and supporting evidence-based practices, we can ensure that herbal medicine continues to thrive and benefit humanity for generations to come.

Chapter 10: Herbal Medicine in Everyday Life

In this chapter, we will explore how herbal medicine can be seamlessly integrated into our daily lives. From simple home remedies to creating herbal first aid kits and using herbs for culinary delights, we'll discover the various ways we can harness the power of plants for improved well-being.

Creating an Herbal Home Apothecary:

Learn how to establish your herbal home apothecary, a collection of essential herbs, tinctures, and remedies to address common ailments. We'll discuss the must-have herbs and tools, storage techniques, and how to prepare and use herbal remedies safely.

Herbal First Aid:

Discover how to use herbs to address minor injuries, burns, cuts, and bruises in your herbal first aid kit. We'll cover herbal antiseptics, wound healing remedies, and soothing balms for quick and effective relief.

Herbal Skincare:

Explore the world of herbal skincare and how to create natural and nourishing beauty products. From herbal facials and skin tonics to herbal-infused oils and body scrubs, we'll reveal the secrets to radiant and healthy skin.

Herbal Culinary Delights:

Herbs not only provide healing benefits but also enhance the flavor of our meals. Learn how to use herbs in cooking to create delicious and nutritious dishes. We'll discuss the best culinary herbs and explore unique recipes that showcase their diverse flavors.

Herbal Teas and Infusions:

Discover the art of making herbal teas and infusions for relaxation, digestion, immune support, and more. We'll explore the benefits of various herbal blends and how to brew the perfect cup of herbal goodness.

Herbal Drinks and Elixirs:

Beyond teas, delve into the world of herbal drinks and elixirs that provide potent health benefits. From herbal tonics and syrups to herbal mocktails and smoothies, we'll explore creative and enjoyable ways to consume medicinal herbs.

Herbal Medicine for Children and Families:

Learn how to safely and effectively use herbal medicine for children's health and well-being. We'll discuss gentle remedies for common childhood ailments and how to involve the whole family in herbal practices.

Herbal Rituals and Sacred Spaces:

Explore the use of herbs in creating sacred spaces and rituals to promote spiritual well-being. From smudging with herbs to herbal baths and meditation practices, we'll discover how herbs can enhance our connection with ourselves and nature.

Herbal Medicine for Pets:

Discover how herbal medicine can benefit our furry companions. We'll explore safe and effective herbal remedies for common pet health issues and how to use herbs to support their overall wellness.

Herbal Gardening and Foraging:

Get practical tips on cultivating your herbal garden and foraging for wild medicinal plants responsibly. We'll discuss the best herbs to grow at home and essential guidelines for ethically harvesting wild herbs.

Herbal Medicine and Self-Care:

Learn how to incorporate herbal medicine into your self-care routine for stress relief, relaxation, and emotional balance. We'll discuss herbal practices that promote self-nurturing and well-being.

Incorporating herbal medicine into our daily lives can be a rewarding and empowering experience. By embracing the natural wisdom of plants and integrating herbal practices into various aspects of our lives, we can enhance our health, connect with nature, and foster a deeper sense of well-being. Let this chapter inspire you to explore the diverse and enchanting world of herbal medicine and its transformative potential in everyday life.

The Future of Herbal Medicine

As we come to the final chapter of this book, we take a glimpse into the future of herbal medicine. The world of natural healing is constantly evolving, and new discoveries and research are expanding our understanding of plant-based remedies. In this chapter, we will explore the emerging trends and potential advancements in herbal medicine, as well as the importance of preserving traditional knowledge and sustainable practices.

Modern Research and Scientific Validation:

We delve into the exciting developments in scientific research on herbal medicine. From clinical trials to pharmacological studies, we'll explore how modern science is validating the efficacy and safety of traditional herbal remedies, paving the way for their integration into mainstream healthcare.

Herbal Medicine in Integrative Health Care:

Discover how herbal medicine is finding its place in integrative health care systems. We'll explore how healthcare professionals are incorporating herbal remedies alongside conventional treatments, offering patients a holistic and personalized approach to healing.

The Rise of Herbal Apothecaries and Herbalists:

Learn about the growing popularity of herbal apothecaries and the resurgence of skilled herbalists. We'll explore the role of these practitioners in guiding individuals on their herbal journey and supporting their health goals.

The Impact of Climate Change on Medicinal Plants:

Climate change poses significant challenges to the availability and sustainability of medicinal plants. We'll discuss the importance of preserving biodiversity, ethical wildcrafting, and cultivating endangered medicinal herbs to protect these invaluable resources for future generations.

Herbal Medicine and Global Health:

Explore the potential of herbal medicine in addressing global health issues. From herbal remedies for infectious diseases to herbal interventions in chronic conditions, we'll discuss how herbal medicine can contribute to improving global health outcomes.

Traditional Wisdom and Cultural Heritage:

Recognizing the rich heritage of herbal medicine, we'll emphasize the significance of preserving traditional knowledge and indigenous practices. We'll explore the importance of respecting cultural wisdom and traditional healing methods passed down through generations.

Herbal Medicine and Personal Empowerment:

We'll delve into how herbal medicine empowers individuals to take charge of their health and well-being. Understanding the principles of self-care and herbal self-reliance, we can foster a deeper connection with nature and our bodies.

The Role of Education and Advocacy:

Explore the importance of education and advocacy in promoting herbal medicine. We'll discuss the need for increased awareness of herbal remedies' benefits and the potential for policy changes to support the integration of herbal medicine into healthcare systems.

The Global Herbal Medicine Movement:

Discover the burgeoning global movement surrounding herbal medicine. From online communities to herbal conferences and workshops, we'll explore how like-minded individuals are coming together to share knowledge, experiences, and ideas.

The Call to Sustainable Practices:

We conclude by highlighting the urgent need for sustainable practices in herbal medicine. Understanding the delicate balance between human needs and nature's offerings, we can make conscious choices to ensure the longevity of herbal traditions.

The future of herbal medicine is promising and holds the potential to transform the way we approach healthcare. As we embrace modern research, integrate herbal practices into conventional medicine, and honor traditional knowledge, we can pave the way for a more holistic and harmonious approach to healing. Let this chapter inspire us to continue exploring the vast world of herbal medicine and contribute to its preservation and evolution for generations to come.

Detoxifying Liver with Alkaline Herbs

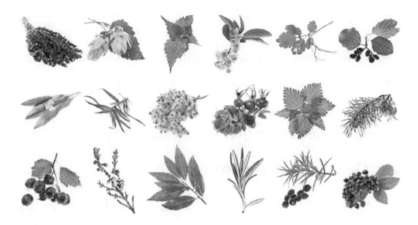

The body contains five organs that clear toxic substances out of the blood circulation and removes them from the system in order to preserve the integrity of the physiological environment for the cells. Your liver, bowels, kidneys, skin (with its sweat and oil glands), and lungs are among these systems.

These detoxing organs, which act as exit gates for toxins in the system, are properly known as eliminatory organs. The cellular environment stays clean whenever these organs are functioning appropriately, and the generation and consumption of contaminants are not excessive. Since the excretory organs eliminate the toxic chemicals at the same pace as they develop, cells may function normally.

You may feel that your medical conditions are unavoidable and that there is little you can do regarding them, yet they are all signs of a liver that is overworked. You can repair your liver by cleaning and purifying it, removing all the impurities, lipids, and pollutants that overload it. It will help you to get clear off of all of your bothersome issues and reclaim your health and vigor. When the number of toxins is too high, however, the organs' eliminative powers are rapidly exhausted, and the cellular environment begins to progressively amass significantly larger concentrations of toxic elements. If the excretory organs are also slow or inadequate, the pace of toxin accumulation will accelerate, resulting in disease.

In this chapter, we'll go through the importance of getting your liver detoxified with medicinal plants and herbs. Then, a subsection will highlight the consequence of having an overworked liver, i.e., all the ailments that an overburdened and slow liver creates for you. Furthermore, we'll also dive into some of the most effective medicinal herbs and herbal teas that can heal and detox your liver if consumed in appropriate amounts.

2.1 Why is Liver Detoxification Important?

In holistic medicine, cleansing of the body as a whole and of the liver especially is of paramount significance. When you understand the concept of terrain, the body's internal ecology, and naturopathic remedies, the usefulness of this therapeutic method will become clearer. For good physical health, there is a perfect terrain makeup that delivers energy and optimum endurance to the body organs. Any change in this makeup damages your wellbeing and renders you prone to sickness, which is a basic result of this desired state of things. Any alteration in the molecular terrain of the system occurs mostly as a result of chemicals that have been introduced to its optimal condition. These are compounds that are either not strange to the environment but are generally present in lesser amounts (uric acid, urea, etc.) or chemicals that do not ordinarily penetrate the terrain's makeup (preservatives, food additives, and so forth). As per natural remedies, the buildup of pollutants that overload the body's internal environment is a major cause of sickness. Overload is at the foundation of the disease, and healing necessitates the removal of these poisons.

Toxins may make us ill in a variety of ways when they build up in the system. Blood thickens, and since it is thicker and denser, it is unable to travel freely through the blood arteries. Wastes that would ordinarily be carried by the circulation to the excretory organs end up in the lymphatic system and other intracellular fluids. The longer this dirty and crowded condition persists, the more these liquids will get polluted. Toxins are detrimental because of their volume, which takes up lots of space that obstructs and blocks arteries and tissues, as well as their hostility, which irritates, inflames, and destroys cells.

Certain toxins in the body are caused by tissue wear and strain. The body must constantly

discard exhausted cells, red blood cell debris; utilize essential minerals, carbon dioxide, nitrogen, and other waste products. The overwhelming majority of toxins are produced through the body's utilization of dietary items. Uric acid and urea are produced by amino acids, lactic acid is produced by sugar, and a range of acids and triglycerides are produced by oils. Toxin generation is natural, and the system is capable of eliminating them. When you eat too much, the quantity of toxins in your body rises much over what is deemed acceptable. Toxic chemicals, on the other hand, should not be present in the body. Toxic chemicals are chemicals that are completely alien to normal bodily functioning and are damaging to the body. Toxic chemicals include all chemical pollutants created by contamination of the atmosphere, food, and land (lead, heavy metals, arsenic, and so on). A considerable amount of dangerous foreign compounds enter the body via typical food supplements, as well as the bulk of insecticides, pesticides, and herbicides used to protect food and livestock goods in modern farming.

Since the body is not built to accept or discharge harmful chemicals, they are hard to remove. If sickness is caused by toxins accumulating in the body, it is only natural that the best treatment would search out and remove these poisons from the body system. Emptying or purging, often known as detox, is a method of removing toxins with the aim of doing so. The liver is the organ most suited to neutralize and remove them because of its cleansing properties. The liver, like the other emunctory systems, is responsible for the elimination of a huge range of poisons. It does, however, neutralize poisons in addition to eliminating them. The other four excretory organs lack this capacity, at least not to the same degree. If they can neutralize poisons at all, it's to a very little degree. Despite the fact that the liver's job is to remove poisons and poisonous chemicals, it may get overburdened by them. As a result, the liver, more than any other excretory organ, must be in top functioning shape. Similarly, when a patient needs to stimulate an excretory organ owing to poor physical function, the liver is usually the most suitable organ. The liver, on the other hand, takes in so much abuse when digesting poisons and poisonous chemicals that it might get overloaded. If this is the situation, and their existence in high amounts is interfering with appropriate liver enzymes, cleansing the liver becomes a primary concern in order to protect the rest of the body's health.

2.2 Ailments Caused by Liver Dysfunction

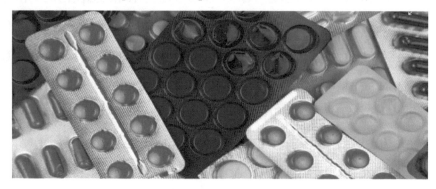

A decrease in liver function may have consequences for systems that aren't even adjacent to the liver. A quick inspection may give the idea that there is no link between the liver and the afflicted systems, but when you consider the function of the environment and chemicals in the pathogenesis of illnesses, the link becomes clear.

1. Gastrointestinal Problems

Liver dysfunction is a common explanation for constipation that is often neglected. A slow liver will not produce sufficient bile, which has the ability to promote gastrointestinal motility, the movement of food particles through the intestine. As a result, not only fiber content but also bile causes the contraction of the gut muscles. Consequently, even if there is a minor deficiency of fiber in the diet, adequate bile production allows the feces to pass through the intestines. The bowels slow down their function when there is a scarcity of bile. The partly digested food becomes stuck and accumulates, making the gut muscles' job more difficult. Constipation will become a problem at this point. Bile also adds moisture, keeping the feces wet and smooth, making passage through the bowels easier. It prevents the feces from sticking to the mucosal surfaces of the intestinal epithelium, which are also slippery due to the presence of bile. This indicates that the stool may simply move forward. Bile deficiency, on the other end, makes feces viscous and impairs motility.

Second, the liver has a variety of functions. Bile emulsifies lipids, breaking them down into small pieces that are then targeted by the pancreatic and gut's digestive fluids. Fatty acids that have not been fully digested can induce uneasiness, bloating, and the very deep feeling that you have not digested your food if this initial step is not done properly. Furthermore, the liver aids digestion by alkalinizing the amount of food traveling through the digestive organs from the previous meal. The stomach produces very acidic digestive fluids in order to break down proteins. The pH of the food as it leaves the stomach is 2.5. The digestive and gastrointestinal fluids that are operative in the bowels, on the other hand, can only be functional in an alkaline atmosphere, i.e., when the pH is greater than 7. The liver is in charge of adjusting the pH of the meal to the level that these digestive fluids need to work efficiently. With a pH that spans from 7.6 to 8.6, the bile it produces is very alkaline. This alkalizes the food, allowing lipids to be digested completely and effectively. However, if a person has liver problems, this alkalizing action will not be enough. Fats will be poorly absorbed, resulting in a range of digestive problems.

2. Cardiovascular Diseases

Heart disease increased blood pressure, cardiac arrest, cerebrovascular disease, and other cardiovascular disorders have many different manifestations, but they all come from the same underlying cause: the buildup of fatty molecules in the circulation. The blood thickens as a result of these compounds, slowing the pace of blood flow. They produce fatty masses in the vessels when they are formed on the walls of blood vessels, diminishing their diameter and limiting blood flow. Blood coagulates when it gets too viscous and sluggish. This clot may obstruct an artery in the heart, causing a cardiac arrest, or in the brain, causing a stroke, or anywhere else in the body, causing an embolism. However, these excess fatty compounds are chemicals that the liver might have blocked from entering the circulation if it hadn't been overburdened by a diet heavy in "poor" fats and sweets. As a result, any therapy for heart disease must include strengthening and purifying the liver.

3. Elevated Cholesterol

All of the fats we eat go straight to the liver. Only a fraction of this amount is used by the system; the rest is converted into triglycerides and cholesterol, which the liver excretes into the bile. This material next enters the bowels, where it is generally expelled with the feces if there is enough fiber (whole grain psyllium husks, natural fibers from fruit and veggies) to catch it. Fiber is necessary for the removal of cholesterol from the body. It's like a perfect trap that catches it. If there isn't enough fiber in the diet, cholesterol isn't bound and is fully absorbed by the system. Up to 90% of cholesterol may be recycled back by the gut wall and returned to the liver if you don't get enough fiber in the diet. The excess cholesterol that is reintroduced to the liver in this manner is not metabolized and removed by this organ but rather enters the overall bloodstream. It builds up in the circulation (metabolic derangement) and forms plaques on the inside of the arteries as a result of the excess amounts. The leading causes of coronary heart disease are blood viscosity and the accumulation of fatty plaques.

4. Metabolic Problems

Low blood sugar strikes certain persons on a regular basis. They experience a rapid loss of strength and vigor, as well as an overpowering sense of tiredness, which is often followed by fainting episodes and dizziness. They are frightened and nervous at times. A shortage of glucose in the bloodstream causes this lack of energy. This leads to strong and frequent cravings for sweet things like chocolate and croissants. Excessive ingestion of poor carbohydrates is the primary cause of hypoglycemia; however, the liver could also be to blame. Blood glucose is "burned" while we go about our everyday routines. Its concentration in the blood decreases, although we are usually unaware of this. The liver, with its infinite wisdom, instantly rectifies and recovers a blood sugar rate that has gone too low. It accomplishes this by unleashing sugar into the circulation, which it has stored in the form of glycogen for this reason. When the liver is exhausted, however, the metabolism of glycogen to sugar is disrupted. As a result, the blood glucose levels drop below standard, and the liver is unable to repair it, resulting in the lack of energy that individuals experience in this condition. Cleansing the liver is, therefore, the cure. It will be able to manage blood glucose levels effectively after it has been healed and strengthened.

2.3 Herbs for Liver Detox

The liver is an important organ in your body since it keeps you clear of toxic substances. It is continually processing waste that enters our system as a result of the atmosphere, nutrition, or poor lifestyle choices. Many additional health issues, including excruciating headaches, persistent exhaustion, hormone issues, nervous system abnormalities, renal problems, hepatitis, cirrhosis, and liver disease, may be caused by a liver that is no longer working effectively. Among the most efficient ways to stimulate liver function is to use herbal remedies. Hepatic plants, often known as liver drainers, are plant species used to cleanse the liver. Each one of these herbs is useful, but their actions differ widely, so it's best to switch plants throughout the duration of a lengthy therapy. This also guarantees that the system doesn't really develop a habit towards a single plant, resulting in a decreased response.

1. Dandelion Root and Leaves

The vivid yellow blossoms of this well-known shrub brighten gardens and pastures. Its tall, serrated leaves give it its name. It promotes all of the liver's processes, including the creation and evacuation of bile, and is regarded as one of the finest herbs with liver-detoxing qualities by many healers. Salads made with dandelion greens are strongly advisable. For generations, the dandelion has been a well-known healing plant. It was common in ancient Egypt, Rome, and Greece, where it was widely used in traditional medicine. Dandelions were most likely brought to North America by migrants seeking therapeutic benefits. Dandelion leaves and roots may be infused for a long time, which enhances its therapeutic effects. Dandelion is a wonderful plant for liver cleaning, despite being a great coffee alternative. You may regain some vitality by detoxifying your liver. As a result, consuming it in the morning is an excellent coffee alternative that permits the whole body to remain in detox mode instead of absorbing all of the acidity that coffee use might produce. This remarkable herb has the potential to boost your immune system, eliminate free radicals, fight diabetes, alleviate nasal problems, and even fight cancer. It also boosts levels of energy, relieves stomach distress, gastrointestinal problems, gallstones, chronic stiffness, muscular pains, and dermatitis, and is used to treat viral infections. It has been used to treat viral infections and boost immunity. It helps reduce inflammation and cholesterol, lowers blood pressure, and aids in glucose homeostasis. Because of its potent antioxidant and anti-inflammatory qualities, dandelion leaf extract benefits the liver. For centuries and centuries, herbal treatments produced from dandelion root and leaves have been used to effectively treat cirrhosis and fatty liver.

2. Artichoke

The leaves of the plant, not the plant's bud, are utilized in treatment. They efficiently but gently promote bile secretion, which explains their reputation as a liver cleanser. Adults and children should consume artichoke leaves in particular. They have diuretic characteristics as well.

3. Garlic

Garlic is a great liver cleanser since it's strong in selenium and allicin. It increases the activity of liver enzymes, making it simpler for the liver to handle and eliminate pollutants. Garlic creates a number of sulfur-containing chemicals that are necessary for the body's nourishment and metabolism. Allicin and selenium, two key elements found in this plant, have been demonstrated to protect the liver from acid toxicity and help it detox.

4. Milk Thistle

The most well-known natural treatment for liver problems is milk thistle. It aids in detoxification, bile synthesis, and liver regeneration. Milk thistle is a herbaceous plant belonging to the Asteraceae family that may be found all around the Mediterranean. Milk thistle is beneficial to liver function because of its antioxidants, anti-inflammatory, cleansing, and regenerative capabilities. It regenerates liver tissues by encouraging the generation of new cells, renewing them, and preserving them from further harm. Its tonic and decongestant effects aid with tiredness, depression, and food intolerances by improving liver function. The silymarin molecule is responsible for the liver's defense. Hepatitis, cirrhosis, drinking, opioids, and environmental contaminants are all absorbed via diet, water, breath, and skin. Thus it's important to get enough of it. It also has galactogenic characteristics since it contains a lot of phytoestrogens, which increases milk production in females. Female hormone synthesis is regulated by phytoestrogens, which is important for a female's overall health.

5. Licorice

Licorice has anti-hepatitis and anti-cancer properties. The licorice root is very useful for liver cleansing. Licorice is a plant that belongs to the bean family and grows as an annual herb. Since olden history, it has been appreciated for culinary and medicinal purposes throughout the Arab World, southwestern Asia, and south of Europe. Licorice's Greek name indicates "sweet root." Other licorice kinds exist, but G. glabra is the most often used in cooking. Licorice is now cultivated all over the Middle East and Central Asia, as well as in mainland Europe and the western United States. Just the roots are utilized, despite the fact that the plant produces little pods with five seeds a piece. When the plants are 3 to 4 years old, they are picked, washed, cut, and dried. Licorice sticks are made from the long segments of the roots (not to be confused with dark black licorice sticks that are actually dried concentrated licorice extract). The leftover roots are cut, diced, or crushed into a powder, and licorice extract is made from them. The powder form of licorice is light brown to grayish-green, with a brown exterior and a light tan inside. When bitten into, the roots have a scent like tobacco— licorice is often used as a flavor component in cigarettes—but produce a pleasant taste that is comparable to fennel or anise. The powder has a strong odor.

Since the Roman era, licorice root has been recommended to relieve sore throats and coughing, chewed for its sweet flavor, and made into a pleasant drink. It is essential in the candy business today, but in most places, particularly India and China, where it was well-known to herbalists hundreds of years ago, its therapeutic qualities have eclipsed its gourmet usage. Sharpened licorice root skewers are occasionally used for grilled steak in Barcelona's Basque area, incorporating it with their taste while it cooks. Alternatively, the roots may be soaked in milk or cream to form an ice cream or custard foundation. Licorice root is an anti-inflammatory that is used in Vedic medicine to treat a number of disorders ranging from digestive discomfort to liver issues, as well as to dental cleanings. Anybody with increased blood pressure, cardiovascular illness, or renal difficulties should avoid it.

6. Chicory Root

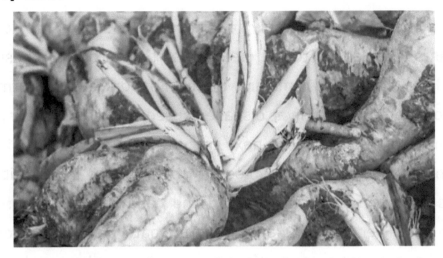

Chicory root has long been used as a traditional treatment for liver problems. It was even utilized by the ancient Egyptians to cleanse both the blood and the liver. It aids in the generation of bile, which aids in the breakdown of fat.

7. Turmeric

Curcumin, one of turmeric's most important components, increases the development of liver detoxifying enzymes. Curcumin also kills cancerous cells in the liver and lowers lipid levels. Turmeric is a tropical root that is related to the ginger family, and the spice originates from the plant's subterranean root systems, much like ginger. It is indigenous to India, and India is still the world's greatest grower and supplier, but it is also extensively cultivated throughout Asia, particularly in Indonesia, as well as in South America and the Caribbean. Entire clusters of turmeric plants are carefully separated from the ground, and the tiny rooted cuttings, known as fingers, are cut off from the bigger roots and cooked or steamed. This procedure speeds up the drying process and prohibits the little clumps from growing. After that, they're dried and cleaned, with the skin removed before being powdered. Because dry roots are very rigid, professional processing is required. The most common kind of powdered turmeric is Madras turmeric, which is a brilliant yellow to orange in color. The Alleppey turmeric is believed to be of superior quality since it is deeper in hue. Both give color to whatever meal they're put to (as well as your fingers, cutting surface, and clothing).

Turmeric makes it considerably quicker for the liver to clear out contaminants when added to the diet. It also boosts bile synthesis (which helps the liver digest food), making the liver's work easier. Turmeric has been demonstrated to heal liver disease caused by alcohol intake, so have some turmeric on board for the next crazy night out. Turmeric is used in herbal remedies and is commonly used to create tea by infusing it with hot water. It's used to help with digestion and ease stomach pain. It's also thought to be a liver tonic and an anti-inflammatory substance for chronic ailments like bronchitis, and it's used as an antibacterial in topical treatments to heal wounds and burns.

8. Blue Vervain

Blue Vervain is a perennial herbaceous plant that grows to a height of 1 meter. Verbena is a European native that favors calcareous grounds. The ability to calm the nerves and muscles is among the most well-known vervain qualities. It comes in handy when you're under a lot of pressure. To get the most out of all of these qualities, brew herbal tea before going to bed. The anticonvulsant and sedative effects of blue vervain are significant. This might open up new possibilities for using this plant to treat neural conditions like seizures in the future. Blue Vervain has a strong anti-inflammatory action, making it useful for treating terrible headaches, migraines, and sinusitis. It's also used to assist the system recover from fevers and illness by facilitating mucus clearance. It has the potential to increase the supply of breast milk in new moms. It also has cardio-protective properties, and its herbal tea, whether drank cold or as a rinse, may help to alleviate periodontal inflammation. Its essential oil possesses antiviral and antibacterial qualities that may help prevent and limit the spread of germs and bacteria, as well as certain forms of fungus.

9. Cascara Sagrada

Cascara sagrada is a tree indigenous to the Pacific coast of the United States, with populations in Chile and California, as well as Europe. Cascara sagrada is a laxative that helps you move your bowels. Based on one's tolerance and problem, it may be taken alone or in combination with other more strong substances like senna. It should only be used in rare situations of severe constipation and in circumstances when simple elimination with softer stools is required, such as hemorrhoids. The bark is very beneficial since it has a mechanical effect on the gut wall, but it should not be used for lengthy periods of time. Cascara should be used no more than twice or three times each week for a maximum of two weeks. Its impact lasts for around 8 hours, so it's best to have it before heading to bed to observe a difference in the morning.

Prolonged use of its essence is not suggested for people with digestive difficulties as well as those living with irritable bowel, liver, heart, or kidney illness since it is an herb that powerfully activates the whole digestive system. Cascara may help with digestion because of its impact on gut motility and fluids. The active compounds in its bark promote liquid and nutritional absorption, as well as liver function and bile evacuation. It's used to treat constipation, hepatitis, liver problems, and cancer, among other things. It's a colon cleanser that's said to improve the colon wall's muscle tone.

10. Yellow Dock

It's indigenous to Asia and Europe, but it's now spread all over the globe, where it's often regarded as a weed. Both the foliage and the roots have medicinal use. Cooking with leaves is also an option. The yellow dock is used medicinally as an extract, syrup, or salve. Yellow dock root tonic is a fantastic treatment for a variety of liver issues. It promotes detoxification and increases the synthesis of bile, which benefits digestion as well as the general health of the liver. Conditions that can be resolved with yellow dock:

- Inadequate digestion
- Liver detox
- Skin disorders (like scabies)

- Inflamed nasal passages

- Rheumatism

- Scurvy

- Constipation

- Promotes bile production\s– In some African countries, warm dock leaves are used to treat inflamed nipples during breastfeeding and also pound and pulp the foliage for use as a piles treatment.

- The dehydrated root of yellow dock combined with hot water is often used as a gargle to cure laryngitis and as a mouth rinse. It is also efficacious against gum disease.

- Bowel infections (like ringworm)\s– Bacteria and fungi infections

- Jaundice

11. Moringa

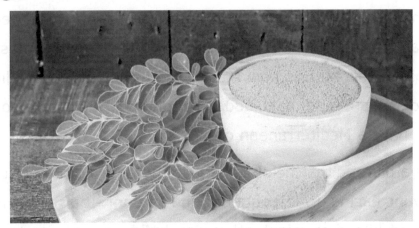

Moringa has been dubbed the "wonder plant" for its many healing properties for decades. It's an all-natural immune booster with a ton of antioxidants. But, probably most importantly, moringa has been demonstrated to be helpful at liver cleansing and boosting liver function, both of which are critical for immune system function. When people's livers are inflamed, their bodies have a hard time getting rid of pollutants, reducing their immunity. Moringa, luckily, is a potent natural anti-inflammatory. Moringa has been investigated for its 40 natural antioxidants and tens of anti-inflammatory substances, which have been shown to help the liver carry out its activities without a hiccup, which is another of the significant moringa liver benefits. Enzymes must be present in full force for your liver to cleanse properly. The enzymes in diseased livers are frequently low or non-existent, preventing detoxification from taking place. Moringa, on the other hand, may stimulate the production of liver enzymes.

12. Boldo

Boldo is a shrub that grows naturally in central Chile and Peru. Boldo is well recognized in the United States as a liver stimulant and for its potential to boost bile secretion. The tea may aid in the treatment of a number of liver and gallbladder problems, including jaundice, hepatitis, and gallstones. The tea may also help with hunger stimulation, digestion, intestinal health, and bloating and constipation relief. Boldo has a distinct, somewhat bitter flavor, which, you all know, is frequently a sign of a food's healing capabilities. It may be consumed on its own or mixed with yerba mate, a famous South

103

American beverage. Boldo's leaves carry all of the plant's therapeutic qualities. They're used to brew tea, a drug-free option that's been around since the dawn of mankind. It was originally used to treat muscular pain and achy joints. This herb is now recognized to help in the healing of liver problems, digestion, and gallbladder problems. Boldo is also found in regions that have a Mediterranean climate.

Boldo tea is a diuretic that helps to reduce the development of uric acid in the blood by increasing urine frequency and amount. It also gets rid of extra salt, fluid, and bile that might otherwise build up and create problems. Peeing on a regular basis may assist in controlling blood pressure, increase hunger, promote digestion, and reduce gas production in the gastrointestinal system. Boldo tea also aids in the treatment of fatty and inflamed livers, as well as cirrhosis, hepatitis, and indigestion. Boldo tea may be used to cure a variety of conditions, including moderate dyspepsia and gastroenteritis. Boldo tea may help boost bile production from the liver during normal working circumstances. As a result, food degradation and metabolic activity in the stomach are accelerated. This guarantees that your food is processed quickly and that the amount of stagnant food in your stomach is reduced. As an outcome, you'll have fewer digestive troubles, including flatulence, cramping, and acidity. Put 1 cup of boiling hot water on 1 teaspoon of dried leaves to prepare boldo drink, steep for 10 to 15 minutes, and take three to four times per day.

2.4 Detoxifying Herbal Teas For Liver

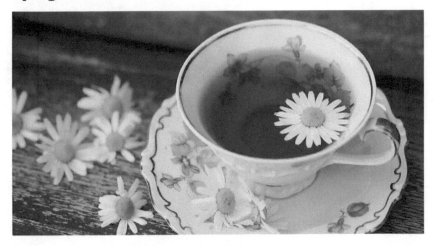

Herbal teas have been utilized as remedies since olden history and for good motives. They're effective. They are plants having delicious and fragrant qualities that are used to enhance dishes, make teas, unwind, or treat medical conditions. Coffee, a booster of the nervous system, tannins having an astringent action, and mineral salts are all found in herbal teas. You are supposed to consume as much water as you like in addition to teas. This aids in the removal of toxic materials from the body and helps you lose weight. Liquids support liver function and, most crucially, increase urination. Try to drink as much freshwater as necessary.

1. Nettle Tea

The stinging nettle, often known as nettle, is a plant native to Northern Europe and Asia. Urtica dioica is its scientific name. The plant has lovely heart-shaped foliage and pink or yellow blooms, but the stalk is coated with small, rigid bristles that, when contacted, emit irritating compounds.

Even though the irritating characteristic of raw nettle is well-known, dehydrated nettle is among the most powerful cleansing herbs. It aids in urinary tract cleaning, and it also includes histamine, which may assist with allergy symptoms. Many plants are beneficial for spring and summer detoxification and reducing clinical manifestations of bodily toxicity; however, nettle is an excellent option for inflammatory dermatitis and allergies, such as coughing and difficulty breathing.

2. Ginger Tea

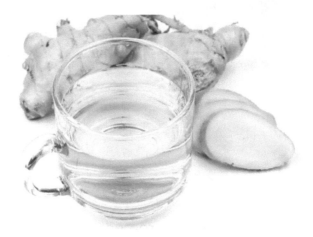

Garlic has huge quantities of allicin and selenium, which are two distinct substances that help detoxify the liver. You may activate liver enzymes that break down and drain toxins in the body by introducing just a tiny bit of this spicy plant to your diet. Though ginger is often referred to as a root, it is really a tuber, the subterranean portion of the ginger plant's stem. Ginger is flexible in addition to having a distinct, enticing taste that is both warm and spicy. It may be prepared in a variety of ways, including fresh, dehydrated, crushed, juiced, or compressed to extract the oil. Healers have employed ginger as a natural treatment for millennia in all of these ways. Ginger is a gastrointestinal remedy that is also supposed to assist with seasickness. Ginger tea may be used to relieve a throat infection or to offer a pleasant, comforting boost, or it can be consumed before traveling.

3. Rosemary Tea

Rosemary is a Mediterranean shrub that blooms on stalks with several tiny thin leaflets that have potent choleretic (can increase bile secretion) and cholagogic characteristics. Because the effects of rosemary are so strong, therapy with this plant should be restricted to one month. Rosemary is also quite energizing and invigorating. Thus it is not suggested for those who are easily agitated. It is highly advised that you utilize it in your meals. To brew the tea, put 1 teaspoon of the leaves in each cup, steep for 15 minutes, and drink two to three cups each day.

4. Horsetail Tea

Horsetail may be found across Asia, North America, and Europe, as well as other parts of the Northern Hemisphere. Horsetail is a one-of-a-kind herb with two different stem kinds. Early in the spring season, one kind of stem emerges, resembling asparagus besides its dark hue and spore-bearing cones on top. The adult version of the plant has branching, thin, green, barren stalks and resembles a fluffy tail when it appears in the summertime. Horsetail has often been used as a diuretic for centuries (helps rid the body of excess fluid by increasing urine output). One research looked at how persons with a background of uric acid kidney disease used horsetail. Horsetail users had more diuresis than those who didn't (urine output). Horsetail contains protective qualities, according to other research, and may suppress cancer cell proliferation.

5. Birch Tea

Birch syrup is used as a traditional treatment in Nordic, Soviet, and Asian societies for strengthening immunity, combating exhaustion, curing arthritis, lowering aches and pains, and minimizing headaches. Birch tree water has also been linked to renal and hepatic cleansing. Tea prepared from the Downy birch (Betula pubescens), which grows abundantly in the Icelandic region, is very healthy and flavorful, making it ideal for everyday use. Birch tea has anti-inflammatory and diuretic properties. Birch is said to help the liver, purify the bloodstream, and treat renal disorders. It's been used to treat bladder infections. Birch is often used to treat rheumatoid arthritis of all types, as well as increasing hypertension and fluid retention development. Saponin, a harsh chemical, resin, polyphenols, tannin, and essential oils are all found in birch leaflets.

6. Bearberry Tea

Bearberry is also known as uva ursi (Arctostaphylos uva ursi). Bearberry's antimicrobial capabilities have been proven to suppress the activity of bacteria such as Escherichia coli and certain other kinds of pathogens, hence guarding against and assisting in the prevention of gastrointestinal illnesses. Because of its strong tannin concentration, it may help with diarrhea and gastroenteritis. The plant Uva Ursi was particularly popular among American Indians, and it was often utilized in ceremonies. Herbal treatment only uses the foliage, not the fruits. It was utilized by American Indians to treat bladder infections. Uva ursi was a typical therapy for bladder infections till the finding of sulfa medicines and penicillin. Soak 3 grams of crushed leaves in 5 oz. of water for Twelve hours to prepare a drink. The drink should then be strained and consumed 3 to 4 times per day.

Chamomile (Matricaria chamomilla)
Medicinal Properties: Chamomile has anti-inflammatory, calming, and digestive properties. It is useful for relieving anxiety, gastrointestinal disorders, and insomnia.

Recipe:

Chamomile Tea for Relaxation:

- Ingredients:

  - 1 tablespoon of chamomile flowers

  - Boiling water

- Instructions:

  1. Pour boiling water over a tablespoon of chamomile flowers.

  2. Steep for 5-10 minutes.

  3. Drink before bedtime to promote sleep.

Sage (Salvia officinalis)

Medicinal Properties: Sage has antibacterial and anti-inflammatory properties and is used to treat sore throats, coughs, and respiratory infections.

Recipe:

Sage Gargle for Sore Throat:

- Ingredients:

  - Sage leaves

  - Boiling water

- Instructions:

  1. Prepare a decoction with sage leaves in boiling water.

  2. Allow it to cool.

  3. Use it for gargling several times a day.

Lavender (Lavandula angustifolia)

Medicinal Properties: Lavender has calming and relaxing properties and is used to alleviate stress, anxiety, and insomnia.

Recipe:

Lavender Essential Oil for Skin Care:

- Ingredients:

  - Lavender essential oil

  - Carrier oil (e.g., olive oil)

- Instructions:

  1. Mix a few drops of lavender essential oil with a carrier oil.

  2. Apply it to the skin to soothe irritations and inflammations.

  3. Ideal for a relaxing bath.

Echinacea (Echinacea purpurea)

Medicinal Properties: Echinacea is known for boosting the immune system and is used for preventing and treating colds and infections.

Recipe:

Echinacea Tincture for Immune Support:

- Ingredients:

  - Echinacea roots

  - Alcohol (for maceration)

- Instructions:

  1. Macerate echinacea roots in alcohol for several weeks.

  2. Use it as a supplement to support the immune system.

Ginseng (Panax ginseng)

Medicinal Properties: Ginseng is a natural tonic that helps improve energy, concentration, and stress resistance.

Recipe:

Ginseng Tea for Energy:

- Ingredients:

  - Ginseng root slices

  - Hot water

- Instructions:

  1. Pour hot water over a few slices of ginseng root.

  2. Steep for 10-15 minutes.

  3. Drink in the morning for a stimulating effect.

Calendula (Calendula officinalis)

Medicinal Properties: Calendula has anti-inflammatory and soothing properties and is used to treat skin irritations and wounds.

Recipe:

Calendula Salve for Skin:

- Ingredients:

  - Calendula flowers

  - Olive oil

- Instructions:

  1. Prepare calendula oil by macerating the flowers in olive oil for several weeks.

  2. Use the oil to make a salve to apply to affected areas.

Peppermint (Mentha x piperita)

Medicinal Properties: Peppermint has digestive properties and can help reduce bloating and stomach discomfort.

Recipe:

Peppermint Tea for Digestion:

- Ingredients:

  - Peppermint leaves

  - Boiling water

- Instructions:

  1. Pour boiling water over a few peppermint leaves.

  2. Steep for 5 minutes.

  3. Drink after meals to aid digestion.

Turmeric (Curcuma longa)

Medicinal Properties: Turmeric has anti-inflammatory and antioxidant properties and is used to alleviate joint pain and inflammation.

Golden Milk with Turmeric:

- Ingredients:

  - Warm almond milk

  - Turmeric powder

  - Black pepper

  - Honey

- Instructions:

  1. Mix warm almond milk with turmeric powder, black pepper, and honey.

  2. Drink to promote joint health.

Recipe:

Aloe Vera (Aloe barbadensis miller)

Medicinal Properties: Aloe vera has soothing properties and is used to treat burns and skin irritations.

Recipe:

DIY Aloe Vera Gel:

- Ingredients:

  - Aloe vera leaf

- Instructions:

  1. Cut an aloe vera leaf and extract the transparent gel.

2. Apply directly to the skin to soothe irritations.

Lemon Balm (Melissa officinalis)

Medicinal Properties: Lemon balm has calming properties and can help reduce anxiety and improve mood.

Recipe:

Lemon Balm Tea for Mental Well-being:

- Ingredients:

  - Lemon balm leaves

  - Hot water

- Instructions:

  1. Pour hot water over a few lemon balm leaves.

  2. Steep for 5-7 minutes.

  3. Drink during moments of stress or agitation.

Guide to Medicinal Plants and Herbs (Continued)

St. John's Wort (Hypericum perforatum)

Medicinal Properties: St. John's Wort is used as a natural antidepressant and mood enhancer.

Recipe: St. John's Wort Infused Oil: Infuse St. John's Wort flowers in olive oil for several weeks. Use the oil topically to alleviate mild depression and nerve pain.

Valerian (Valeriana officinalis)

Medicinal Properties: Valerian is known for its sedative properties and is used to promote sleep and alleviate anxiety.

Recipe: Valerian Root Sleep Aid: Prepare a decoction with valerian root in water and drink before bedtime for a restful sleep.

Dandelion (Taraxacum officinale)

Medicinal Properties: Dandelion has diuretic properties and is used to support liver and kidney health.

Recipe: Dandelion Detox Tea: Steep dandelion leaves and roots in hot water for 10 minutes. Drink to help cleanse the body.

Elderberry (Sambucus nigra)

Medicinal Properties: Elderberry is known for its immune-boosting properties and is used to prevent and treat colds and flu.

Recipe: Elderberry Syrup for Immune Support: Boil elderberries in water, strain, and add honey. Take as a daily supplement during cold and flu season.

Garlic (Allium sativum)

Medicinal Properties: Garlic has antimicrobial properties and is used to boost the immune system and support heart health.

Recipe: Garlic Honey for Immunity: Crush garlic cloves and mix them with honey. Consume a teaspoon daily to enhance immunity.

Rosemary (Rosmarinus officinalis)

Medicinal Properties: Rosemary has antioxidant and anti-inflammatory properties and is used to improve cognitive function and digestion.

Recipe: Rosemary Oil for Hair and Scalp: Infuse rosemary leaves in olive oil for several weeks. Use the oil as a hair and scalp treatment.

Yarrow (Achillea millefolium)

Medicinal Properties: Yarrow has astringent and anti-inflammatory properties and is used to treat wounds and minor bleeding.

Recipe: Yarrow Salve for Wound Healing: Prepare a salve using yarrow-infused oil and beeswax. Apply to wounds for healing.

Nettle (Urtica dioica)

Medicinal Properties: Nettle is a natural anti-allergen and is used to alleviate seasonal allergies and hay fever.

Recipe: Nettle Leaf Tea for Allergies: Steep nettle leaves in hot water for 5 minutes. Drink to relieve allergy symptoms.

Licorice (Glycyrrhiza glabra)

Medicinal Properties: Licorice has anti-inflammatory properties and is used to soothe sore throats and digestive issues.

Recipe: Licorice Root Tea for Digestive Health: Boil licorice root in water and steep for 10 minutes. Drink to relieve digestive discomfort.

Ginger (Zingiber officinale)

Medicinal Properties: Ginger has anti-nausea and anti-inflammatory properties and is used to alleviate nausea and muscle pain.

Recipe: Ginger Infused Water for Nausea: Infuse ginger slices in water and drink to ease nausea and indigestion.

Creating Herbal Formulations

In this chapter, we will delve into the art of creating herbal formulations by combining various medicinal plants and herbs to enhance their healing properties. Formulations can be in the form of teas, tinctures, salves, oils, and more, each serving specific health purposes. Understanding the synergy between different herbs will allow you to create potent and effective remedies for various ailments.

Herbal Tea Blends

Exploring the art of herbal tea blending and how to combine different herbs to address specific health concerns.

Recipes for Relaxing Herbal Tea, Immune-Boosting Tea, Digestive Aid Tea, and more.

Herbal Tinctures and Extracts

Understanding the process of making herbal tinctures and extracts using alcohol or glycerin as solvents.

Recipes for Calming Tincture, Energy-Boosting Tincture, and Immune Support Extract.

Herbal Salves and Balms

Discovering the process of creating healing salves and balms using infused oils and beeswax.

Recipes for Healing Salve for Cuts and Scrapes, Muscle Relief Balm, and Skin Soothing Salve.

Herbal Oils and Infused Vinegars

Exploring the benefits of herbal oils and vinegars and how to create them for culinary and medicinal use.

Recipes for Herbal-Infused Olive Oil, Rosemary-Infused Vinegar, and Lavender-Infused Sunflower Oil.

Herbal Capsules and Pills

Learning how to encapsulate powdered herbs for convenient and controlled dosing.

Recipes for Herbal Sleep Aid Capsules, Immune Support Pills, and Digestive Health Capsules.

Herbal Medicine for Special Populations

In this chapter, we will discuss the considerations for using herbal medicine for special populations, including children, pregnant individuals, and the elderly. Understanding the appropriate herbs and dosages for these groups is crucial to ensure their safety and efficacy.

Herbal Remedies for Children

Exploring gentle and safe herbs suitable for children's specific health needs.

Recipes for Calming Herbal Syrup for Kids, Immune-Boosting Gummies, and Soothing Herbal Teething Rub.

Herbal Support during Pregnancy

Understanding which herbs are safe to use during pregnancy and which ones to avoid.

Recipes for Nausea-Relief Herbal Tea for Pregnant Women, Pregnancy-Safe Herbal Baths, and Postpartum Healing Salve.

Herbal Care for the Elderly

Addressing common health concerns in the elderly and herbal remedies for improved well-being.

Recipes for Memory and Cognitive Support Tincture, Joint Pain Relief Herbal Oil, and Energy-Boosting Herbal Tea for Seniors.

Chapter 12: Harvesting and Storing Medicinal Herbs

Restoring Health with Medicinal Herbs

Harvesting Medicinal Herbs

Understanding the best time and methods for harvesting different parts of the plant.

Tips for drying, freezing, and preserving fresh herbs.

Storing Medicinal Herbs

Learning how to store dried herbs properly to maintain their quality.

Creating a home herbal apothecary and organizing your herbal collection.

Safety and Precautions in Herbal Medicine

In this chapter, we will emphasize the importance of safety and precautions when using herbal medicine. Understanding potential interactions, contraindications, and proper dosages is vital to ensure the well-being of those using herbal remedies.

Herb-Drug Interactions

Exploring potential interactions between herbal remedies and conventional medications.

Highlighting common herb-drug interactions and how to avoid them.

Allergic Reactions and Contraindications

Identifying herbs that may cause allergic reactions or contraindications for certain individuals.

Educating readers on how to recognize and avoid adverse reactions.

Dosage Guidelines and Proper Usage

Providing clear dosage guidelines for each herb and formulation discussed in the book.

Emphasizing the importance of following recommended dosages for safe usage.

Integrating Herbal Medicine with Conventional Healthcare

In this final chapter, we will explore the integration of herbal medicine with conventional healthcare. Understanding the role of herbal medicine as complementary to modern medical treatments will empower readers to make informed decisions about their health and well-being.

Collaboration with Healthcare Professionals

Encouraging open communication with healthcare providers when incorporating herbal medicine into a treatment plan.

Highlighting the benefits of an integrative approach to healthcare.

Holistic Approach to Health

Emphasizing the importance of addressing the physical, emotional, and spiritual aspects of health for overall well-being.

Exploring the concept of holistic healing and its role in herbal medicine.

In the concluding section, we will summarize the key takeaways from the book and reinforce the power of herbal medicine in promoting natural healing and overall wellness. We will encourage readers to continue exploring the world of medicinal plants and herbs to embark on their journey toward becoming knowledgeable and confident herbalists.

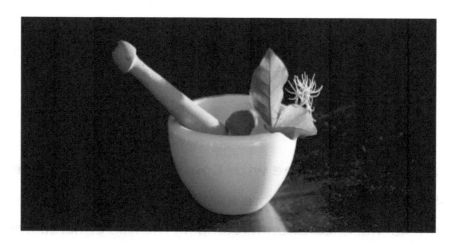

There are three illnesses we'll talk about in this chapter, i.e., pancreas, kidneys and intestinal problems. First of all, kidney stones are made up of waste products — substances that the body doesn't need. This waste is usually excreted in urine by your kidneys. If there is excess waste or there isn't sufficient water to wash it all out, it becomes a stone. These stones can be so tiny that they resemble sand or grains. The agony that these crystals cause when they are removed by the kidney may be terrible. It is frequently likened negatively to labor or anesthesia-free operation. Medical research can't explain for sure why some individuals are more susceptible to stone formation than others. However, they do run in generations, implying a hereditary susceptibility to the illness. Prolonged dehydration has also been linked to some forms of disordered eating. Kidney stones affect around one in every 15 individuals in the developed world nowadays. In certain areas, that figure is as high as one in five. Every year, upwards of a million Americans are admitted to hospitals for treatment of the disease.

And what was previously primarily a male condition now impacts many females as well.

Similarly, the pancreas is another one of our very important organs, as it helps in the production of bile which helps in digesting fats and other foods. If the pancreas is not working properly due to eating a diet full of processed, acidic foods, you will start developing gastrointestinal problems like irritable bowel syndrome. Hence, the pancreas and intestines are infinitely linked with each other. So, detoxifying and healing them with natural medicinal herbs is essential for optimal health, which is what this chapter entails.

3.1 Herbs for Pancreatic Health

The pancreas is a digestive organ that generates hormones and digestive enzymes. People who have diabetes, in particular, rely on it to operate properly. Several herbs, luckily, not only preserve the pancreatic tissues against illness but also aid in its restoration if it becomes swollen, as in the instance of pancreatitis.

1. Licorice Root

The root and subterranean roots of the perennial herb called Glycyrrhiza glabra are known as licorice roots. Licorice's anti-inflammatory qualities may help alleviate the discomfort and edema associated with pancreatitis. Licorice is a good ancient treatment for decreasing inflammation of the respiratory system since it possesses antimicrobial, antibacterial, purgative, and anti-inflammatory effects. Tea, pills, and extract are all options. This plant works well in a combining solution with other plants. Licorice root has been used as a flavor enhancer, confectionery uses, and therapeutic reasons by the Greeks, Egyptians, Asians, as well as other Eastern civilizations for ages.

2. Echinacea

The numerous echinacea plants have been utilized by native groups in North America for a long period of time. The nine species of Echinacea may be utilized, but the most frequently seem to be Echinacea Angustifolia and Echinacea purpurea. Echinacea, which is strong in antioxidants, is an effective natural therapy for a variety of airway problems (e.g., bronchitis). The root extract and raw liquid of the airborne plant are by far the most effective therapeutic forms of the herb. It's used as a complementary treatment in Germany for common cold, persistent infections of the bronchial and lower urinary system, and topically for sores that don't heal well and persistent ulcers. Its root extract is combined with other botanicals to treat influenza-like symptoms.

3. Oregano

Oregano is an effective natural therapy for high glucose levels and many other diabetes-related problems. It also offers plenty of amazing health advantages. Antioxidants including vitamins A, C, as well as vitamin K are abundant in Mediterranean oregano. Essential oregano oil is used to treat a range of diseases, and its tea may be made to relieve coughing and upset stomachs. In the Greek region, there are several distinct types, which are generally known as rigani.

4. Garlic

Garlic is beneficial to the pancreas since it lowers blood glucose levels while also stimulating insulin production in the pancreatic tissues. The kidneys are yet another vital organ for your general wellbeing. Their major job is filtering blood, which they accomplish by eliminating waste products from the system (mainly urea). They also control the amount of water and salt in the system. Progressive kidney disease, or decrease of kidney function over time, is a life-threatening disorder. Unfortunately, many individuals are completely ignorant that their kidneys are progressively deteriorating. High blood sugar and blood pressure are the primary causes of this illness.

5. Olive Leaf Extract

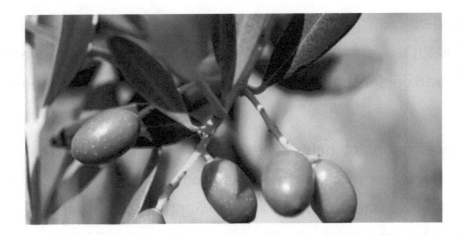

The pancreas will operate better if you utilize olive leaves extract (herbal extract) on a regular basis. It also relieves the discomfort and edema associated with pancreatitis and shields the pancreas from oxidative stress induced by free radicals. Your chances of pancreatic cancer will be greatly reduced if you utilize it on a regular basis.

6. Lemons

Lemons are chockfull of vitamin C and magnesium, giving a dietary boost to pancreatitis sufferers.

7. Goldenseal

Hydrastis Canadensis is the scientific name, while goldenseal has been the most popular choice. Indigenous Americans have long used it to cure skin illnesses, gastrointestinal issues, liver problems, dysentery, and eye infections. This plant is very good for diabetes patients since it aids the pancreas by reducing blood glucose levels. Its herbal medication is made from dehydrated roots. Because it is a superb organic plant that supports glowing skin, goldenseal extract is often incorporated into a variety of skin and beauty products. Goldenseal is used to treat the flu virus and also various upper respiratory infections, congested noses, and seasonal allergies. Goldenseal is used to treat stomach discomfort and inflammation (gastritis), gastric sores, anal ulcers, colitis (intestinal inflammation), diarrhea, stomach cramps, hemorrhoids, and extreme flatulence in certain individuals. Goldenseal is available in a variety of forms, including pills, powdered, extract, and drink.

The goldenseal root, particularly when combined with Echinacea, provides several health advantages. One of the most important advantages of Echinacea and goldenseal would be that they support the immune system.

8. Gentian

Gentian root treatment helps digestion by increasing pancreatic enzyme synthesis. Hot water mixed with gentian root has also been used to relieve edema in the liver, stomach, and spleen. Gentian root is derived from plant species of the Gentiana genus, which comprises over 400 species found in the mountains of Europe, Asia, and North America. Gentian blooms appear in a range of lovely hues. However, the root is really the only part of the plant that is utilized medicinally. It's golden in color and may be processed for tablets, infusions, extracts, and tinctures. People typically combine it with water and use it externally or consume it in herbal medicine. Decrease in hunger, bloating, intestinal gas, indigestion, gastritis, acid reflux, and puking are all treated with gentian. Fever, hysteria, and excessive blood pressure are also treated with it. Gentian is used to avoid muscular cramps, cure intestinal parasites, initiate menstrual cycles, and fight pathogens, among other things.

3.2 Herbs for Kidney Health

Dr. Sebi believed in two simple but strong principles for kidney's wellbeing: drink enough water and get rid of mucus and pollutants. You must drink sufficient liquids to make up for all other deficits while still having enough to neutralize pee. In terms of toxins, changing the things that have a negative influence on your system on a daily basis will affect the makeup of your urine. A rise in what individuals ingest has been linked to kidney stones. We must cope with more junk as our meals become more diversified. Waste passes via the kidneys and is excreted as urine. Let's look at the herbs and medicinal plants you can take for curing as well as preventing kidney disease.

1. Horsetail

It is prized for its diuretic effects, which aid in the elimination of waste from the urinary system and bladder. To manufacture medication, just the portions of the herb that are above the surface are utilized. Horsetail is used to treat "water retention" (puffiness), kidney and urethra stones, bladder infections, leakage (incapability to regulate urine), and overall kidney and bladder problems. The kidneys struggle hard to clear contaminants and control urine; horsetail may aid in this process by removing uric acid, which forms kidney stones. There is a strong link between ingesting horsetail and having reduced uric acid concentrations in the body, excess of which ultimately creates kidney stones. Baldness, hepatitis, cirrhosis, fragile nails, joint problems, arthritis, rheumatism, bone disease (reduced bone density), hypothermia, loss of weight, intense menstrual cycles, and profuse bleeding (severe bleeding) of the nasal passage, chest, or gut are also treated with it.

2. Green Tea

It is suggested to those whose kidney function is not in optimal condition because of its potent anti-inflammatory and hypotensive qualities. It also comprises antioxidants, which aim to minimize kidney stones from forming. Green tea includes catechins, which are a type of flavonoids that seem to suppress infectious diseases by attaching to the virus and thereby blocking the pathogen from reaching the host tissues. It comes in the form of tea bags or dried leaves. To make the tea, combine 20 ounces of green tea leaves with 6 ounces of water. Green tea may also be consumed as a pill or capsule three to four times each day. Consume no more than 5 cups of green tea each day.

3. Hydrangea Root

This herb is excellent for urinary and renal function. Restricts kidney stones from developing by assisting the body in using calcium so that there isn't an excess that the tissue will convert to kidney stones.

4. Couch Grass

The plant will boost your kidney output (peeing), which can help you cure any of the urinary tract infections simply since the more and more you pee, the more microbes you will clear out. Couch grass may also aid in the removal of kidney stones.

5. Goldenrod

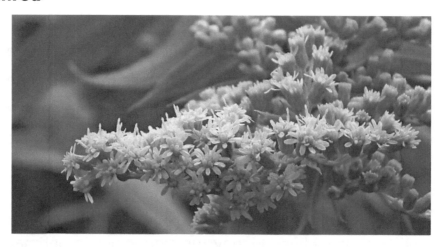

Goldenrod, which is also known as Solidago canadensis, has traditionally been used to treat sores on the body. It's also been used as a purgative, which means it aids in the removal of surplus water from the system. In Europe, it's used to cure urinary tract infections and kidney problems, as well as to minimize or cure them. Goldenrod is often used in infusions to assist in washing away kidney stones and prevent urinary tract illnesses. "To make complete" is the meaning of the term solidago. It's a long-used treatment for bladder and kidneys and renal ailments in general. Goldenrod is sometimes used as "irrigation treatment." This is a treatment that entails consuming goldenrod with plenty of water to enhance the flow of urine in order to cure chronic conditions of the lower urinary tract and also kidney and urinary tract stones. Its usage as a bladder and kidneys health defender is also supported by new research.

6. Chanca Piedra

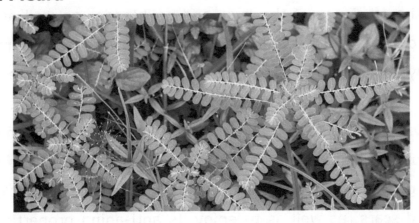

Chanca piedra often referred to as "stone buster," is a medicinal herb that is supposed to be a miracle cure for kidney disease. Chanca piedra is a Phyllanthaceae family annual herb. The plant may be found in the Amazon jungle as well as in other tropical climates across the globe. An herbal remedy made from the whole plant is utilized as infusions, pills, liquid solutions, and capsules. Gout recurrences are caused by the growth of uric acid in the vascular system, which also causes kidney stones. Chanca piedra has been proven to help regulate this excessive production of uric acid and avoid painful gout episodes. The plant is said to help with ulceration, kidney and bladder stones, and a variety of disorders involving the kidneys, liver, and gastrointestinal tract. When it relates to effectively removing kidney stones, it's the most popular plant in South America. Chanca piedra got its name from its usefulness as a renal stone remedy. The herb's alkaline qualities may aid in the prevention of gallbladder and toxic kidney stones.

7. Java Tea

Drinking Java tea would not only enable you to keep your kidneys functional, but it will also certainly assist you in disintegrating kidney stones and healing renal infections.

8. Dandelion

Dandelion root is a powerful cleanser and an excellent herbal renal detoxifier. Dandelion is a popular blooming plant that grows all across the globe and is prized for both its roots and blooms. As a diuretic and purgative, dandelion is commonly used with the burdock plant to treat gastrointestinal diseases. It relieves upset stomach and gas while also improving the efficiency of the liver and gallbladder as well as intestinal health. Its diuretic effect is mild on the body due to its mineral content, which partly refills the amount lost via peeing, allowing the person to maintain a healthy alkaline equilibrium. It may help ladies with fluid retention. Dandelion is also great for the cure of urinary tract infections and kidney problems. Its anti-inflammatory properties aid healing while also safeguarding renal function. It may be used on the skin to treat dermatitis, wounds, and scars, as well as to enjoy its anti-aging properties. It helps with skin pigmentation problems. Finally, it aids in blood sugar management, making it a viable alternative for diabetics.

9. Celery Root

Both the root and the seeds are diuretic and should be used by anybody who has urinary tract issues.

3.3 Herbs for Intestinal Detox (Colon Cleanse)

Colon cleansing is a term used to describe the process of removing waste from the intestines. For hundreds of years, it has been a common practice. But, while an intestinal detox has numerous advantages, it also has some drawbacks. Herbs in the shape of brews, pills, or powders are a substitute for colon cleansing in a facility. Many plants are anti-inflammatory and function as herbal laxatives.

1. Cascara Sagrada

Cascara sagrada is a plant indigenous to the Pacific coast of the United States, with populations in Chile and California, as well as Europe. Its skin is the most helpful component, and it is so potent that it requires a year after collecting to nearly fully eliminate the side effects of its usage. After that year, it may be used for a variety of ailments without causing stomach discomfort, vomiting, or diarrhea. It's a mild laxative that helps you move your bowels. Based on one's tolerance and problem, it may be taken alone or in combination with other more strong substances like senna. It should only be used in rare situations of severe constipation and in circumstances when simple elimination with soft stools is required, like hemorrhoids.

The bark is very beneficial since it has a mechanical effect on the gut wall, but it should not be used for lengthy periods of time. Cascara should be used not any more than twice or three times each week for a maximum of 15 days. Its impact lasts for around eight hours, so it's best to apply it before getting in bed to observe a difference in the morning. Excessive use of its extract is not suggested for anyone with digestive difficulties or even those living with irritable bowel, liver, cardiovascular, or renal problems since it is an herb that powerfully activates the whole digestion process. Cascara may help with digestion because of its impact on gut motility and hydration. The active compounds in its bark promote liquid and nutritional uptake, as well as liver function and bile output. It usually causes a bowel movement within ten to 12 hours. Therefore it's wise to take it at nighttime so you can use the toilet more easily in the morning.

2. Senna
Senna tea or pills are a strong laxative that shouldn't be taken for any more than a couple of days at a time.

3. Rhubarb Root
The word "rhubarb" originated from the Latin word "rhabarbarum." The roots of Rhabarbarum were employed as a cleanser by the Chinese as way back as five thousand years ago. Rhubarb is an herb that is indigenous to Asia and Europe which is now grown all over the globe. For generations, its root has also been used to treat many ailments. It's harvested when the plant is about a year old, dried, and used in tiny pieces or powdered, mostly in teas. Rhubarb root is taken as a laxative, as well as to enhance liver function and digestion. Since it has a strong impact on your bowels, it is important to keep its usage to a minimum in terms of amount and regularity. Rhubarb root includes numerous chemicals that assist digestion by activating the gall bladder and cleansing the blood by removing heavy

metals. It also helps in the detoxification of toxic chemicals and dangerous microorganisms from the intestine. Constipation, gas, and cramping may all be relieved with this supplement.

4. Psyllium Husk

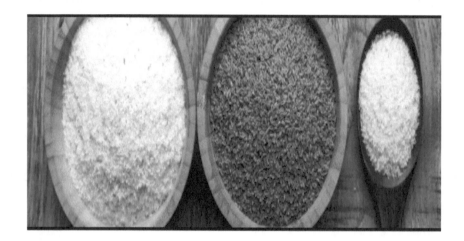

Psyllium seeds and husk are a very well-recognized colon cleaning folk medicine. The presence of mucilage, a form of fiber that absorbs moisture in the gastrointestinal tract, is what gives it such an effective laxative effect.

5. Fennel

Fennel is a fragrant plant indigenous to the Mediterranean region that comes from the Umbelliferae family and has the scientific name Foeniculum Vulgare Miller. Fennel is primarily used as a fragrant plant, but it also offers a wide range of health advantages. Purifying and gastrointestinal herbal teas may be made using leaves and seeds. The seeds, in particular, are high in active substances, which are beneficial to the biological mechanisms of the gastrointestinal tract. Its crude extract is likewise high in estrogen-like chemicals. It is often used in conjunction with laxatives, such as rhubarb or senna. It's gentle to administer to kids on its own. It also has an antispasmodic action, which aids in the elimination of unpleasant digestive colic in infants, and is ideal for individuals experiencing abdominal discomfort as a result of digestive problems.

Fennel is a diuretic that aids in the removal of excess bodily fluids. Its cleansing characteristics make it even better when combined with other alkaline plants, including dandelion root and milk thistle. Fennel tea has several health advantages, particularly for individuals who suffer from digestion problems such as stomach ache, abdominal discomfort, stomach pain with contractions, and gastritis with reflux may all profit greatly from a decent cup of fennel tea, which can be consumed following dinners or throughout the day to cleanse the stomach. Fennel improves stool motion, removes excess gas, sanitizes the colon, and relieves cramping and aches in cases of gastrointestinal abnormalities, inflammatory bowel disease, constipation, diarrhea, spasms.

Fennel has a purgative effect, which helps to clear and remove mucus. In the night, a warm infusion promotes respiration and helps you get a good night's sleep.

6. Barberry Bark

This plant promotes bile production and works as a natural laxative, which benefits intestinal function.

7. Black Walnut

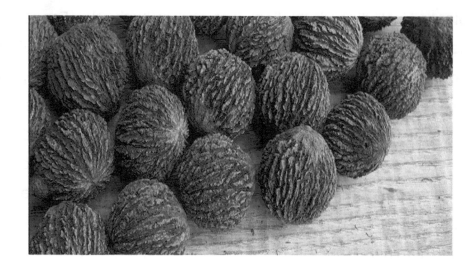

Juglans nigra is the official name for the tree, which is predominantly found in the United States of America. The seed is the only part of the plant that may be eaten. They're a potent natural vermifuge and are used to fight intestinal worms that may harm people. Candida Albicans is a fungal pathogen in our intestines. Consuming black walnuts will improve our intestinal health and help Candida Albicans' life as difficult as possible.

In this chapter, we will discuss the art of harvesting and storing medicinal herbs to preserve their potency and freshness for extended use.

VIDEO COURSE

Conclusion

Embracing Herbal Wellness

As we journey through the pages of this comprehensive guide, we've embarked on a path of discovery, empowerment, and connection with the natural world. The diverse realms of herbal medicine, plant cultivation, and crafting remedies have been unveiled, revealing the boundless potential of nature's gifts.

In this concluding chapter, let's take a moment to reflect on the remarkable journey we've undertaken together. From the foundational understanding of herbal medicine to the intricate art of cultivating healing plants, we've delved into the rich tapestry of botanical healing.

Throughout this book, we've explored the wisdom of traditional herbalism, uncovering the secrets held by ancient cultures and indigenous knowledge. We've navigated the realm of essential oils, discovering their potent aromas and therapeutic applications. We've embarked on the intricate process of crafting tinctures, infusions, and salves, unlocking the alchemical transformation of plants into powerful remedies.

As we conclude this journey, remember that our connection to nature's remedies is a lifelong partnership. The knowledge and skills you've gained here are but the beginning. With each seed sown, each herb harvested, and each remedy created, you contribute to your own well-being and that of those around you.

Embrace the ongoing journey of herbal wellness, for it's a journey that intertwines you with the very essence of life itself. By cultivating healing herbs and harnessing their potential, you become a steward of ancient traditions, a seeker of natural balance, and a conduit for the healing energy of the earth.

Let this book be your guiding companion on this ongoing adventure. May the wisdom of plants continue to enrich your life, nurturing your body, mind, and spirit. As you walk the path of herbal wellness, remember that you are not merely an observer but an active participant in the intricate dance of nature's healing magic.

With heartfelt gratitude for joining us on this journey, we bid you farewell, knowing that the world of herbal wellness is now at your fingertips. As you venture forth, may the spirit of healing plants be your constant guide, and may the vibrant energy of nature infuse every step you take.

Wishing you a life of vibrant health, abundant knowledge, and harmonious connection with the world of herbal remedies.

Blessings on your herbal journey